YOUR BODY AFTER THE BIRTH

Jane Chumbley is a freelance health writer who specializes in pregnancy and early parenting. She is a practising antenatal teacher with the National Childbirth Trust (NCT) and has two young sons.

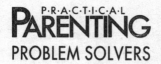

PROBLEM SOLVERS

YOUR BODY AFTER THE BIRTH

JANE CHUMBLEY

PAN BOOKS

First published 1999 by Pan Books

an imprint of Macmillan Publishers Ltd
25 Eccleston Place, London SW1W 9NF
and Basingstoke

Associated companies throughout the world

ISBN 0 330 37049 9

Copyright © Jane Chumbley 1999

The right of Jane Chumbley to be identified as the
author of this work has been asserted by her in accordance
with the Copyright, Designs and Patents Act 1988.

Illustrations by Debbie Hinks except
pages 47, 81, 82 by Raymond Turvey

All rights reserved. No part of this publication may be
reproduced, stored in or introduced into a retrieval system, or
transmitted, in any form, or by any means (electronic, mechanical,
photocopying, recording or otherwise) without the prior written
permission of the publisher. Any person who does any unauthorized
act in relation to this publication may be liable to criminal
prosecution and civil claims for damages.

1 3 5 7 9 8 6 4 2

A CIP catalogue record for this book is available from
the British Library.

Typeset by SetSystems Ltd, Saffron Walden, Essex
Printed and bound in Great Britain by
Mackays of Chatham plc, Chatham, Kent

This book is sold subject to the condition that it shall not,
by way of trade or otherwise, be lent, re-sold, hired out,
or otherwise circulated without the publisher's prior consent
in any form of binding or cover other than that in which
it is published and without a similar condition including this
condition being imposed on the subsequent purchaser.

Practical Parenting is published monthly by the SouthBank Publishing Group,
IPC Magazines Ltd, King's Reach Tower, Stamford Street, London SE1 9LS.
For subscription enquiries and overseas orders call 01444-445555 (fax no 01444-445599).
Please send orders, address changes and all correspondence to: IPC Magazines Ltd,
Oakfield House, 35 Perrymount Road, Haywards Heath, West Sussex RH16 3DH.
Alternatively, you can call the subscriptions credit card hotline (UK orders only) on 01622 778778.

Contents

Acknowledgements vii

Introduction ix

PART ONE: EARLY DAYS

1 **What's happening down below?** 4

2 **Breast changes** 18

3 **After a Caesarean** 28

PART TWO: MOVING ON

4 **Getting back to normal?** 40

5 **Pelvic floor** 47

6 **Weight and shape** 56

Contents

7 **Backache** 79

8 **Other joints, aches and pains** 98

9 **Sex** 106

10 **Skin and hair** 117

11 **Tiredness** 121

12 **What about my hormones?** 129

Further information 145

Acknowledgements

Thank you to all the women who were so very generous in giving me their time and were willing to talk so openly about their experiences.

Introduction

The days, weeks and months after you give birth are precious. The last things you want are physical or emotional problems which will prevent you from enjoying your baby. This book has been written to help you solve any problems which may arise. Sometimes the solution lies in your own hands; sometimes you'll need to ask for professional help. At all times, it helps to understand the nature of the problem – why it may have occurred in the first place – and to know that you aren't alone. One thing you'll soon discover – if you haven't already – is that everyone you meet has a tale to tell and a piece of advice to give. Sometimes that's great and just what you need, but there are lots of old wives' tales and handed-down wisdom – how do you know who is right? Research trials tell us about what works for most women, but you aren't most women! You're an individual. And in some cases, the detailed research simply hasn't been done. So sometimes, to a certain extent, you have to accept that it's trial and error: every woman is different and different things seem to work for different people. This book offers you lots of ideas to try out and opportunities to find something that works for you.

Part One

EARLY DAYS

'I was completely shell-shocked. I just kept thinking over and over again: how is it no one told me about this? You put a brave face on it, and of course you're very happy about the baby, but I felt I just needed three weeks off to recover!'

Giving birth is rarely like shelling peas – whatever your granny might have told you. Even if you have a fairly quick, relatively painless birth with no tears or stitches, your body still has to recover from being pregnant and undo the work of nine months, as well as get you ready for breastfeeding – whether you intend to or not!

The first few days after your baby is born can be a very confusing time. You want to spend time enjoying your baby and you want to put her first, but things are happening to your body and you may feel you have no control over them. If you don't know what to expect, perfectly normal things like blood loss or after-pains can be very frightening.

The following chapters describe some of the things that can happen in these very early days – the first ten days of your baby's life – and there are lots of suggestions for ways you can help yourself. Part Two focuses on longer-term problems.

1
What's happening down below?

Blood loss

When the placenta detaches from the wall of your womb it leaves behind a raw patch which bleeds. This blood loss – called lochia – is like a very heavy period for the first twelve hours, then starts to reduce, but the bleeding can go on for some weeks as the raw patch heals and is gradually covered with the endometrium – the normal womb lining. The lochia change colour over this time, from bright red in the first week to pale pink or brown for the next couple of weeks or so. After that, some women have a creamy-white vaginal discharge, possibly for another month. If you pass a clot of blood bigger than a 10p piece you should tell your midwife – this can be a sign that part of the placenta has been left behind.

Bleeding like this isn't much fun, particularly when you're coping with the demands of a new baby. You can make it easier to cope with, though, by being well prepared:

- Buy several packs of the largest sanitary towels you can find – either maternity pads or the overnight ones. Change your pad

What's happening down below?

every time you go to the toilet and don't switch to smaller pads until you are sure the blood loss is tailing off.
- Think about your knickers. Some women prefer to wear disposable knickers for the first week or so, and the advantage of these is obvious – you'll have less messy washing and won't stain your best underwear if you leak over a pad. But disposable knickers aren't always that comfortable and some brands tear easily: if you're keen to use them, buy one pack and try them before spending a lot of money. NCT Maternity Sales* sell washable high-waisted stretch briefs which may be a better option, particularly after a Caesarean (see page 28). Alternatively, dig out those baggy old knickers from the back of your underwear drawer and use them instead.
- Find an old towel or terry nappy and a plastic sheet to protect your mattress from blood leaks in the night.

When is blood loss not normal?

- When it contains clots – especially if you are in pain as well.
- When it goes on for more than six weeks.
- When it smells – this can be a sign of infection.
- When it is suddenly very heavy and continues to be heavy – this can be a sign of haemorrhage (called a secondary postpartum haemorrhage): get help straightaway.

Q&A

I was really pleased when I stopped bleeding after only ten days but then a day or two later I had a sudden rush of red blood again. Why?
Some women find that they start bleeding heavily again when they become more active after having a baby, because walking

---

* Indicates that further information is supplied at the end of the book.

around drains the lochia. Unless the blood loss is continuously heavy or contains clots there's no danger. Some women find they get a sudden loss of blood when they breastfeed: this is because breastfeeding releases a hormone called oxytocin, the same hormone that made your womb contract in labour (see After-pains below).

Should I be taking iron tablets to stop me getting anaemic?
Not unless they are recommended by your doctor. Normal blood loss after you've had a baby shouldn't leave you anaemic, but if you feel very weak, breathless and faint, tell your midwife: it's very easy to have a blood test to check your haemoglobin level (see page 124).

After-pains

It's not entirely clear what makes your womb shrink back to its pre-pregnant size after the baby is born, but some women are aware they are having occasional contractions even days after the birth, and these may be part of the process. These so-called 'after-pains' can be anything from a dull ache like a mild period pain to something like a full-blown contraction. They often come as you breastfeed and last for perhaps five or ten minutes. This is because breastfeeding releases the hormone oxytocin, which produced contractions in labour. Very occasionally after-pains occur when the womb is trying to push out a clot, so it's worth mentioning them to your midwife (see 'Blood loss', page 5). After-pains normally stop after four days. In the meantime you can:

What's happening down below?

- Take paracetamol twenty to thirty minutes before you begin breastfeeding, but don't exceed the maximum dose.
- Use the relaxation techniques and calm breathing that helped you during labour.
- Tell your midwife – especially if the pains are very severe.

If your abdomen is tender to touch this may be a sign of infection, so tell your midwife when she examines you.

Most textbooks will tell you that few first-time mothers have after-pains and that they are more common after second babies. But there are no hard-and-fast rules.

> Lucy had after-pains following the births of both her sons: 'They started the day after I had my first baby. I went to the hospital loo and collapsed in absolute agony. The pain was excruciating and I was terrified. The midwife gave me Ponstan 40 (a strong painkiller) which was brilliant, and I had a prescription to come home with because the pain lasted a few days. It was just as bad when I had my second baby but at least I knew what to expect. It's the last thing you need when you think you've got over the birth!'

> Emma had to call out the doctor on the fourth day after her first child was born, because her after-pains were so bad: 'He prescribed some painkillers but basically I was dreading every feed because that brought on the cramps. I was in floods of tears, it was so bad. When I had my second child I was expecting the same thing but there was nothing – I didn't feel a thing!'

Your body after the birth

Q&A

I didn't have any after-pains with my first baby: how come they're so bad with my second?
There are various theories about this. One possible explanation is that pains are mostly the result of small areas of scar tissue in the womb left after the previous pregnancy. Some women do have after-pains following their first pregnancy but it's twice as common to have them after a second, third or fourth.

Going to the toilet

Unless you've had an elective Caesarean, and whether or not you've had stitches, it's quite likely you'll have tiny tears, grazes or bruises around your vagina and perineum (the skin between your anus and the entrance to your vagina). These grazes swell as they heal and can feel sore or sting when you pass water. If your perineum is bruised and swollen it may feel numb and strange when you try to pass water for the first time. What's more, pressure from the baby during the pushing stage of labour can cause bruising and swelling in the urinary tract, which will make it more painful to urinate.

If passing water does hurt, you may be tempted to cut back on drinks or delay going to the toilet. But fluids help to prevent constipation which can hurt even more (see 'Constipation', page 10), a full bladder can stop your womb shrinking to its pre-pregnant size, and retaining urine can lead to infection (see below). So:

What's happening down below?

- Go to the toilet as soon as you can after having the baby.
- If you find it difficult to start urinating because you are afraid it will hurt, turn on the taps; the sound of running water can help to relax your muscles.
- Keep a jug or a thoroughly cleaned squeezy bottle in the bathroom. Fill it with warm water and pour or squeeze the water over your stitches as you urinate. This dilutes the urine and makes it less likely to sting.
- Sit well back on the toilet seat and tilt your bottom so that the urine is more likely to go straight into the toilet and less likely to drizzle over your sore area.
- Pass water when you are in the bath and then wash yourself down or shower afterwards.

Urine infection

The symptoms of urinary tract infection are needing to go frequently, pain when you pee, smelly urine and a high temperature. Urine infections are fairly common after childbirth, mainly because of changes in your body brought about by pregnancy. It takes about six weeks for these changes to sort themselves out, so an infection is possible all that time. The treatment depends on the type of infection but could be potassium citrate mixture (available from the chemist) or antibiotics from your doctor. Drinking large amounts of water – at least 3 litres (5¼ pints) a day – will help to prevent an infection and flush it out of your system if you do get one. You can also help to prevent urinary tract infection by going to the toilet frequently and making sure you empty your bladder completely each time.

Constipation

Constipation is actually a side-effect of pregnancy: it's the result of high levels of the hormone progesterone slowing your bowels down, and this can carry on for a few days after you deliver your baby. But some women become constipated after labour because they are worried their stitches will burst if they open their bowels. This kind of anxiety is quite normal and there's no absolute need to go to the toilet in the first day or two. But after a while faeces can build up and lead to problems, so it's a good idea to try.

- Eat plenty of high-fibre foods after delivery – wholemeal bread, bran-rich cereal, figs and prunes, for example.
- Drink water during labour and afterwards.
- If you are worried about your stitches, protect them by holding a clean sanitary towel against your genital area as you push, to relieve any pressure.
- Don't strain. If you feel yourself tensing up through anxiety, use the relaxed, calm breathing you used in labour.
- If you can't go and you feel constipated, ask your doctor for a suppository or lactulose (a laxative).
- If you're in hospital, go home as soon as you can! Using your own toilet may be the only cure you need.

Piles

Like constipation, piles are fairly common during pregnancy because progesterone relaxes your veins and the blood tends to pool. For the same reason you may have had varicose veins in

What's happening down below?

your legs while you were pregnant. But piles (haemorrhoids) can appear for the first time after you've given birth because straining in the pushing stage of labour can stretch the blood vessels in the anus. The resulting piles can be incredibly itchy, painful and uncomfortable. Pregnancy piles nearly always disappear within three months but they should go quicker if you use a pile-shrinking ointment or cream. If you have piles which bleed a lot there's a slight risk you could become anaemic, so mention any bleeding to your GP.

- Make sure you have plenty of fibre in your diet to avoid constipation (see above).
- Use warm water or moist tissues to wipe yourself after you've been to the toilet.
- Wear loose cotton underwear and avoid tight jeans.
- An ice-pack or a moist cotton pad can be soothing if the piles are very itchy.
- Ask your GP to prescribe a pile-shrinking ointment which will also help with the itching. Alternatively, ask the pharmacist for a cream you can buy.

Janet describes how she spent a happy week in hospital after her first child was born: *'So when I did go home I was happy and feeling confident. I didn't expect any more pain, but that wasn't to be! I remember sitting in our breakfast room to breastfeed Daniel and finding the pain coming from my tail end almost unbearable. I even remember saying to my husband, "The pain I have now is worse than giving birth." I thought it was from the stitches and it would go. My husband supplied me with ice packs for a few days until I couldn't bear it any longer; the pain just wasn't going away. So I asked the health visitor to take a look and see if it was all healing as it should. "My dear, you've got piles!" she said – which totally shocked and humiliated me as I thought they were something old men got! Once they were diagnosed it didn't take long for the doctor to treat me and I was soon fine. I suppose that's what you get from all that pushing! I had suffered from varicose veins from the age of twenty-four so I suppose there was already a weakness there.'*

Rose had piles throughout her first pregnancy and afterwards, but even she wasn't prepared for what happened after her second child was born: *'It was day two, and a huge plum-like pile appeared! Apparently it broke some record with the midwives! The consultant tried to replace it, which was incredibly painful and meant I needed pethidine – which I hadn't needed even during labour. A surgeon even came to talk to me about what would be involved in having it removed but I wasn't keen on that. In the end I had to use a Valley Cushion (see below) for six weeks. I was given a cream and suppositories and put on a high-fibre diet and gradually it shrank and disappeared.'*

Stress incontinence

When you overcome any difficulties in starting to pass water, you may find it's actually hard to stop. That's not surprising when you consider how the muscles in your pelvis, including the ring of muscles around your urethra (the duct which lets urine out), have been stretched in childbirth. If you find you wet yourself when you laugh, cough or sneeze, you are suffering from stress incontinence. It's very common in the first year after childbirth – particularly if you have a forceps delivery which may bruise or stretch your muscles. So:

- Restart pelvic floor exercises as soon as possible after you've given birth – within hours if you can (see page 47).
- Don't panic if you can't stop the flow of urine when you first go to the toilet – it's bound to take a bit of time for the muscles to get back into shape.
- Empty your bladder as often as you can.

Stress incontinence during pregnancy is caused by the increasing weight of the baby and the relaxing effect of the hormone progesterone on your pelvic floor muscles. Once you've had your baby, the amount of progesterone in your body drops rapidly, so you should be able to start getting your muscle tone back quite quickly. Ask your GP to refer you to a physiotherapist for help if stress incontinence goes on for more than a couple of months (see page 48).

Stitches and episiotomies

If you have stitches to repair a tear or an episiotomy you may feel quite sore for the first week and it may be difficult to sit down or feel relaxed when you are sitting. Brisk walks will be out of the question! But your perineum is amazingly resilient, and things should start to feel better after a few days. Meanwhile, there's a lot you can do to promote healing and make yourself more comfortable.

- Sit on a Valley Cushion – an inflatable cushion with a dip in the middle – it won't put any pressure on your sore area. Ask

Your body after the birth

if there is one at the hospital, or you can hire one from your local branch of the National Childbirth Trust.* (Rubber rings aren't the same as they restrict blood flow.)
- When you're awake in bed, lie propped up on your side.
- Use a pad of tissues to dry your stitches after a bath. If you want to use a towel, make sure it is soft, keep it just for your genital area and avoid rubbing.
- If you are in hospital, either take showers or get your partner to clean the bath thoroughly before you use it, as stitches can become infected quite easily.
- Apply an ice pack (or wrapped-up bag of frozen peas) to the sore area for short-term relief.
- If you are in a lot of pain, take paracetamol or ibuprofen or ask your midwife if you can use a lignocaine anaesthetic gel or spray.
- Camomile or lavender oil in your bath may help bring down the swelling.
- Being upright and mobile will also help the swelling and bruising to heal more quickly.
- Start doing pelvic floor exercises as soon as you can (see page 47): some research has found that this could help to reduce inflammation and pain.
- If the stitches start to feel tight after a few days (because the tissues have swollen) your midwife can snip them to relieve the pressure.
- Arnica (tablets) and comfrey (tablets or tea) are thought to help with bruising. If you are interested in using homeopathic or herbal remedies it makes sense to consult a registered practitioner.* You could do this before the birth.
- Ask for help if your perineum still feels very sore after a week: you may have an infection.

What's happening down below?

Caroline had an episiotomy when her baby Lucy was born: *'I had a lot of pain from stitches – more than I thought I'd have. In fact, I was in agony. I remember having real problems going to the loo and one day when my mum was here I crawled back into the lounge on my knees crying with pain. I said, "I never knew it would be so painful," and she said, "I don't think it's meant to be." When I talked to the midwife on about day eight or nine she said the stitches were too tight and she cut them, but that turned out to be more painful than giving birth. It just isn't fair, is it? I thought I'd been through enough. Now Lucy's seven months old and I do feel I'm back to normal.'*

Joan had a second-degree tear when her son Timothy was born: *'The stitching was done very quickly and painlessly but over the next few days it was very difficult to sit comfortably. The stitches were a bit like barbed wire. Even walking was uncomfortable as the sanitary towel seemed to rub on them. I remember the relief when one fell out and I got the midwife to snip one of the others. Fortunately it healed in less than ten days, although at the time you don't know that and it feels like for ever!'*

Julia had an episiotomy when her son Guy was born: She explains how she also had an epidural so she was quite numb for most of the day: *'The next day it was like being knocked over by a steamroller! The episiotomy was painful every time I went to the toilet although it was okay walking as long as I didn't rush. What helped most was kneeling rather than sitting in the bath, and I used lavender oil in the bathwater which was very soothing. I also used cypress oil which seemed to help the healing. I was advised to sit on bags of frozen peas but I found that very uncomfortable. It was better lying on one side and applying an ice pack. The Valley Cushion I hired from the NCT was a tremendous help, especially when I was feeding. I suppose it was about ten weeks before I felt I'd got back to normal.'*

Q&A

Will I have to have the stitches taken out?
Not necessarily. Stitches are often done with soluble thread, so they never have to be removed – they just dissolve. Sometimes a stitch may fall out after a couple of days, and your midwife will be able to judge whether the tear is healing properly without it.

Should I put salt in the bath to help healing?
Research shows that adding salt or disinfectant to bathwater does not help healing. By contrast, adding lavender oil to the bath three to five days after birth has been found to reduce discomfort without any side-effects. Lavender oil is antiseptic.

Someone told me witch hazel helps with soreness – is that right?
Some people (including some doctors and midwives) do recommend using gauze pads soaked in witch hazel but research suggests the witch hazel is no more effective than tap water.

No stitches for me please!

These days midwives are happier to leave first- or even second-degree tears to heal on their own without stitches. Something to look forward to next time!

What's happening down below?

Thrombosis

Anyone who spends a few days or more in bed is at risk of thrombosis – a blood clot in the leg. The symptoms are a red, tender or painful patch on the leg and possibly swelling and a high temperature. A thrombosis can be fatal: in some cases the blood clot can move to the lungs. So make sure you report any of the above symptoms to your midwife. You can help prevent thrombosis by getting up and about as soon as possible after you have your baby, and by doing ankle-circling exercises when you are resting.

2
Breast changes

Breasts were designed for feeding babies. So it's not surprising that there are some changes once you've actually given birth to the baby who needs food. However, breasts are also sexual and an important part of our self-image, so some women have very mixed feelings about these changes – particularly if there are problems. Understanding what is happening may help you to cope with these feelings and encourage you to sit back and enjoy giving your baby the most perfect food possible.

Engorgement

About three or four days after your baby is born your breasts will start to swell. This is caused by a surge in the milk-producing hormone prolactin which increases the blood supply to your breasts so that the ducts open and are ready to produce milk (not the yellow colostrum that your baby gets in the first few days). Sometimes, though, breasts become so swollen that they feel hot, hard and painful, as if they're about to explode.

Engorgement is painful and lasts for a day or two, but it shouldn't produce any long-term problems unless your baby

Breast changes

isn't in quite the right position for feeding and isn't draining the breast properly.

- Feed your baby as often as possible.
- Make sure your baby is in the right position (see box on page 25). Get help if necessary. Ask your midwife to spend time with you as you feed, or contact a breastfeeding counsellor from the National Childbirth Trust,* La Leche League,* the Association of Breastfeeding Mothers* or the Breastfeeding Network.*
- Wear a front-opening or drop-cup feeding bra which has been fitted by a trained fitter (the local branch of the National Childbirth Trust* may have a MAVA bra agent who can arrange a fitting for you).
- Relax in a warm bath and gently smooth the flat of your hand against your breasts to express a little milk.
- A warm shower on your breasts may encourage some milk to flow and provide relief.
- Put cold flannels on your breasts between feeds.
- Place chilled Savoy cabbage leaves inside your bra: these are thought to contain an enzyme which may relieve the engorgement.

If your breasts are so full that the baby can't latch on properly, there's a risk your nipples might become sore (see below) or that you might develop a blocked duct.

Sore nipples

Most first-time mums say their nipples feel slightly tender when they start to breastfeed. But sore nipples are not inevitable. If

Your body after the birth

your baby is in the right position she should be taking most of the areola – the pink/brown area surrounding the nipple – into her mouth, and the nipples shouldn't get sore. If they do get red, sore, cracked and even blistered there's almost certainly a positioning problem, with the baby sucking the nipple rather than milking the breast. Nipples can also get sore if you pull the baby off the breast during a feed, or if your baby has thrush (a fungal infection) in her mouth. The most likely time for sore nipples is during the first week, after your milk has come in.

- Get help with positioning (see box, page 25). A pillow under the baby or a different position, such as the American football hold (with the baby's body tucked under your arm), may be the answer for you: everyone's breasts are a different shape.
- At the end of a feed, gently insert your little finger into your baby's mouth to unlatch. Express a little milk and let it dry on to the nipple: breast milk is thought to have healing properties.
- Let your nipples dry in the air.
- Change breast pads regularly so that your nipples don't get soggy between feeds.
- Apply ice wrapped in a flannel to your nipples before feeding, as an anaesthetic.
- If your nipples are cracked and feeding is very painful, use a thin latex nipple shield, available from pharmacists. Many women say these are lifesavers, although shields may make feeds take longer and can reduce your milk supply if you go on using them. (And some babies don't like them.) Try them for one day to see how you get on.
- Don't restrict feeds, but feed on the least sore side first.
- Check your baby's mouth for signs of thrush (white patches in the mouth) and if necessary see your GP for a prescription. Untreated thrush can lead to infective mastitis (see page 22).

Blocked ducts

Inside your breasts there is a network of ducts bringing milk from milk-producing cells to the nipple. If one of these ducts gets blocked (because the milk isn't being drained from it), you may feel hot and shivery and find a hot, tender red patch on one of your breasts. Getting the milk flowing will unblock the duct and the red patch should disappear within a few days.

- Don't stop feeding from the lumpy breast – that will only make the problem worse.
- Check that your bra isn't too tight or that you aren't putting any pressure on your breasts during a feed (by holding the breast, for example, or using breast shells – cups that collect milk drops).
- Feed from the lumpy breast first while your baby is really hungry and sucking strongly. Let her empty the breast fully before you switch to the other side.
- If your breast still feels lumpy after a feed, get some more milk out by hand, using a wide-toothed comb dipped in baby oil. Stroke the comb *gently* towards your nipple to help the milk flow.
- Gently massage the lumpy breast towards the nipple while you are in the bath.
- Use hot or cold flannels or a hot-water bottle to ease the pain.
- If you have a high temperature or flu-like symptoms, you may have mastitis (see below).

Mastitis

The symptoms of mastitis are the same as those for a blocked duct (see above) but the hot, shivery feeling is much more like flu. Mastitis is caused by milk leaking from a blocked duct into the bloodstream where it is treated as a foreign substance, creating swelling and inflammation. That doesn't mean you have an infection or that your breastmilk is infected. Most mastitis is non-infective. Following the advice for a blocked duct given above may solve the problem. If the problem hasn't gone after twenty-four hours, see your GP.

Infective mastitis is the result of bacteria getting into the breast, perhaps through a crack in the nipple. In this case you will need antibiotics. You may need to point out to the doctor that you are breastfeeding (incredible though this may sound!) and ask for an antibiotic you can take while you carry on feeding. Rest as much as you can.

> **If you have the symptoms of mastitis and you spot any blood or pus in your milk, see your doctor straightaway: you may have a breast abscess which needs to be lanced. You can continue feeding on the other side.**

Q&A

A friend of mine used a special cream when she had sore nipples – is it any good?
Breastfeeding experts usually advise women not to bother with creams: there is no evidence from trials that they work. If you use something other than a herbal cream such as Kamillosan you will need to wash it off before you feed your baby. Herbal creams can be left on unless the taste seems to bother the baby.

Why do I keep getting sore red lumps on my breasts?
These are probably blocked ducts (see above). Perhaps your bra is too tight, or are you holding your breast when you feed? Or are you using breast shells to collect drips? Any pressure on the duct system inside the breast could stop the milk flowing and cause a blockage.

Why do I find breastfeeding so painful?
If there are no obvious problems such as cracked nipples, it's possible the pain could be caused by a powerful 'let-down' reflex as the milk cells in the breast contract and push out milk. This usually only lasts for the first week or two but it can be agony. Paracetamol will help to dull the pain. Alternatively, it could be caused by thrush in the milk ducts. If this is the case you may see white spots on the nipple and in your baby's mouth. You may also feel your breasts throbbing between feeds. Check with your GP who can prescribe an antifungal treatment suitable for you and your baby.

Why haven't I got enough milk for my one-month-old baby? She sucks really strongly and at the end of a feed there's nothing left, but she always seems hungry for more.

Breastfeeding works on the principle of supply and demand, or rather, demand and supply, so the more your baby demands, the more milk you produce. It's possible that your baby is having a growth spurt, though, in which case it will take a few days for your milk supply to catch up with her needs. The important thing is to keep feeding: if you stop, your milk supply will reduce. One idea is to let your baby empty one breast, then transfer her to the other while the first breast is refilling. Experts say an hour is long enough to refill the breast completely but the refilling starts immediately. If your baby seems particularly hungry in the evening, try expressing a bottle of milk in the morning to use as a top-up in the evening. That way you'll be stimulating your breasts to produce more milk and giving yourself a rest. Eat and drink well and get plenty of rest.

My breasts keep changing size and I can't seem to get it right with bras. When should you buy them? While you're pregnant, when your breasts are biggest, or afterwards, when they've settled down?

There are two issues here: the size of your breasts and the size of your ribcage which expands in pregnancy. When you're thirty-six weeks pregnant your ribcage should have expanded to its maximum so that's a good time to have a fitting with someone who is properly trained in fitting feeding bras. Some women find that their breasts change a lot over the first few weeks, but a well-fitted bra is designed to cope with a bit of expansion and contraction. However, if your daytime bra just can't cope with the size of your breasts when the milk first comes in, wear a fitted night bra for a few days. Night bras provide light support but they're not restricting and you can go on using them at night even when your breasts have settled down.

> **Good positioning**
>
> If your baby is in a good position for feeding you can avoid or correct the problems of sore nipples, blocked ducts and poor milk supply.
>
> - Sit comfortably and upright.
> - Hold your baby so that her face is towards your breast: she shouldn't have her neck twisted. Line her nose up with your nipple so that when she opens her mouth she has to lift her chin.
> - Stroke her cheek with your nipple or finger: she should then open her mouth wide.
> - Bring your baby to the breast (not the breast to the baby).
> - Your baby should take all the nipple and most of the areola into her mouth.
> - Look for her nose being close to or even touching your breast; the muscle behind her ear moving as she swallows.
>
> If you have any doubt about the way to position your baby, put your little finger into the side of her mouth to break the suction and ASK FOR HELP to reposition her before soreness becomes a problem.

Your body after the birth

When Caroline had her first baby she wasn't anticipating any problems: *'I had a really straightforward birth and you expect to feel great afterwards, so I was completely knocked sideways when I had trouble breastfeeding. He just wasn't latching on properly, and by the second day I had sore nipples. They were so sore I couldn't believe it. Everything hurt and I hated wearing anything. Then my breasts filled up and went rock-hard and I got mastitis. But the NCT breastfeeding counsellor who came to see me was really positive and supportive. She had lots of ideas and really kept me going. What seemed to work best was freezing a flannel, or putting ice cubes inside a flannel, and holding it on the nipples before feeding. That deadened the pain a bit and once he was feeding well from me I felt much more confident. It also helped that Stephen, my husband, was supportive. He stood up to the midwives who suggested I give Richard bottles. You expect it to work instantly, but it doesn't with all babies. I think we just got off on the wrong track, but in the end I breastfed him very happily for over a year. When I had Alexandra she had very similar problems latching on – I think there's just a lot of me to latch on to and they've only got small mouths! It took her about a week to get the hang of it but this time I was much more relaxed and I didn't force her on – or let the midwives force her on – so I didn't get sore.'*

Julie found breastfeeding very straightforward but says it was hard to come to terms with her changing shape: *'I couldn't believe how big my breasts became. They'd got bigger while I was pregnant but when I had them measured about five or six days after I'd had Robin I was a 42D!*

Breast changes

That's a lot for someone who used to be a 34B. I felt really top-heavy and actually found it very hard to cope with how I felt about myself. I felt really clumsy and I kept thinking people must be looking at me. I think my husband thought it was a bit odd too: I just wasn't myself somehow and I hated it if anyone took any photos of me. I thought about giving up breastfeeding but it seemed such a trivial reason when several of my friends had really sore nipples. After a while I just got used to it – and then it was a shock when I stopped feeding and they went back to normal!'

3
After a Caesarean

In practical terms, whether you give birth vaginally or by Caesarean you may experience many of the same things – blood loss, after-pains, engorged breasts and sore nipples, for example (see Chapters 1 and 2). You may also experience some stress incontinence, because even though the perineum hasn't been stretched in labour – unless you have a very late emergency section – the pelvic floor muscles have had to support a considerable increase in weight during pregnancy and have been subject to the same relaxing hormones (see Chapter 5).

But Caesarean section is a major abdominal operation, so there are other after-effects, and your body will almost certainly need more time to recover. After all, if you'd had a hernia operation you'd be off work for up to three months.

Moving around

For the first few days any kind of movement can be difficult because so much of what we do involves the abdominal muscles which are parted in a Caesarean. So it may be hard getting out of bed, standing, walking and lifting. You will need help with your own washing and dressing, and with your baby. There's no reason at all why you shouldn't breastfeed, but you will need someone to pick up the baby and get her in a good position. A physiotherapist should help you to find a comfortable way to cough and sneeze – both can be difficult in the first few days, again because they involve the abdominal muscles.

On the mend: tips for coping

- Ask for help whenever you want to get up or hold your baby.
- Try to get up as soon as you can – within a few hours if possible. This helps to get your circulation moving and prevents blood clots from developing.
- Use calm breathing to help you relax as you move. Go at your own pace and support the scar with your hand if you find that helpful.
- Wriggle your toes and circle your ankles while you are in bed to keep the circulation going (see Thrombosis below). It can also help you move wind in your abdomen.
- Lay a pillow across your stomach to support your baby while you feed her. Alternatively you could tuck her body under your arm like an American football or lie on your side to feed. Get a breastfeeding counsellor* to help you with positioning. Have a shower when your partner can be with you to help with drying and dressing. Ask if you can have a chair in the shower to sit on.
- Keep a pack of wet wipes by your bed so you can freshen up without going to the bathroom.
- Get some slip-on slippers so you don't have to bend down to put them on.

Your body after the birth

- Wear waist-high pants to avoid anything rubbing on the wound. NCT Maternity Sales* sell special washable stretch briefs which are ideal for this.
- Put a pillow between you and the seat belt when you go home and whenever you are in a car.
- Get someone to do all the housework and shopping for you for at least the first month.
- You won't be able to drive or do any heavy lifting for about four to six weeks.

Thrombosis

A thombosis is a blood clot in the leg (see page 17). There are two types — one serious, one not — but both can be caused by poor circulation. Anyone who spends a long time in bed after having a baby is at risk, whether the birth has been Caesarean or vaginal. In the first type — thrombophlebitis — the clot usually forms in a varicose vein. It feels tender and looks red. Special support stockings will help, as will getting up and about, and the pain should go after a couple of days. In the second type — deep vein thrombosis — there may be pain, swelling and a rise in temperature. The danger is that the clot will move to the lungs, so you should be watched closely and given drugs to prevent further clots.

You can help to prevent thrombosis by getting up and about as soon as possible (ideally within six hours of giving birth) and increasing the amount you walk about each day. If your legs are swollen or painful, tell a midwife.

Pain

The amount of pain women feel after a Caesarean – and where they feel it – varies a lot. You may experience pain in your stomach, your arm (where the drip was in place), your back (if you had an epidural) or your throat (if you had a general anaesthetic). The important thing is to make sure you get enough pain relief. In other words, don't just grit your teeth. There are several options – injections, tablets or a top-up to an epidural if you have one in place. The pain around the scar usually goes after a couple of weeks.

Stitches and infections

The dressing on the wound is normally left in place for a couple of days and the stitches (or clips) removed if necessary after about five days. This can be uncomfortable but isn't necessarily painful. The scar usually feels more comfortable afterwards, especially if the stitches were a bit tight. However, about one in five women will get an infection in the wound simply because there are bacteria in the air. If this happens, your temperature will rise, the scar will become red and weepy, and you'll be given antibiotics. Some hospitals give antibiotics to every woman who has a Caesarean to prevent infections (these will be compatible with breastfeeding).

Wind and constipation

Having a rumbly tummy and passing lots of wind is common for up to forty-eight hours after a section. It's the direct result of the operation when air is trapped in your abdomen. It's fairly

Your body after the birth

unlikely you'll open your bowels for a few days because the operation makes your bowel sluggish.

- Avoid fizzy drinks, including mineral water.
- Ask the midwife for some peppermint water and get your partner to buy you some fennel tea.
- If after a few days you feel constipated, ask the midwife for a laxative.
- When you do go to the toilet, support the scar with your hand and try to relax, using calm breathing.

Itching

The scar may start to itch as it heals, as will any regrowth of pubic hair that was shaved before the Caesarean. It may help to:

- Keep wearing high-waisted pants (see box on page 30).
- Use a soothing cream, such as Calendula, or talcum powder on the itchy area.

Exercises

Ideally, every woman having a Caesarean should see an obstetric physiotherapist for advice on exercising. But some hospitals have cut back on these services and you may just be given an exercise sheet or – worse still – nothing at all. It is important you don't try to do too much but also that you do try to do something! In the first days while you are still in hospital do:

- Ankle circling – ten on each ankle, whenever you think of it.
- Foot pedalling – bending your foot towards you and then stretching it away, again in sets of ten per foot.
- Pelvic floor exercises (see page 49).

When you feel ready to try something for your abdominal muscles, check with your midwife and get her to be there when you try. Start with:

- Pelvic tilting – on your back, knees bent, feet flat on the bed. Breathe out as you pull in your abdominal muscles and squeeze your lower back into the bed. You should feel your pelvis tilt upwards as you do this. Hold briefly and release. Repeat in sets of three or four about three times a day.
- Leg sliding – as for pelvic tilting, but slide one leg down the bed as you pull in your abdominal muscles. If your back arches off the bed, stop. As your muscles get stronger you should be able to get your legs out straight. Repeat whenever you think of it!

Q&A

My scar is still painful four weeks after I had the Caesarean. My doctor said it wasn't infected but could there be something wrong?
Although most women say the scar stops being painful after a couple of weeks it is not unheard of for the pain to go on for longer. One study found that one in five women had some pain even three months after the birth. If your scar is still painful at your six- or eight-week postnatal check, mention it again to your doctor and ask him at what point he would organize a test to check everything is healing properly. In the meantime, look out for signs of infection (redness, weeping and the pain getting worse).

I can feel lumps around my scar – is that normal?
It's quite common to feel these lumps. Usually they are bruises caused by slight bleeding under the skin and they will heal in time.

In a couple of places around my scar it feels really numb. Will the sensation come back?
Yes, it should come back over the next couple of months. The numbness is caused by small nerves which have been cut during the operation.

I feel so miserable. I just want to cry all the time.
This is a common and very normal reaction to surgery which is probably made worse by all the hormonal changes going on in your body (see page 129) and any disappointment or anger you feel about having the Caesarean in the first place. It may help to talk to someone who has been through the same experience, someone who really understands. Your local branch of the National Childbirth Trust* may have a Caesarean Support Group with women who are prepared to listen. Don't let people convince you that your feelings aren't important: hopefully they will pass within a few days or weeks, but at the moment they are very real and you need the chance to talk about them. You may also find it helpful to read more about Caesareans.*

I am terrified I am going to hurt myself every time I try to do something. Sometimes I have nightmares that the scar splits and I'm starting to bleed. Is this normal?
It's perfectly normal to be scared you'll hurt yourself: you've had major surgery and it takes time to recover. Having someone with you to hold your arm and talk to you while you move about will help a lot, as will calm, relaxed breathing: breathe in through your nose and out – slowly – through your mouth. Nightmares after an operation are not unheard of, and they will probably stop as you start to recover physically and you're able to give more attention to your baby. But do talk to your GP or

one of the staff at the hospital. If you're still having nightmares after a couple of weeks it might help to have some counselling (which your GP can organize for you).

I had the most terrible headache after my Caesarean. Was it because of the anaesthetic?
Quite possibly, yes. Headaches are a recognized side-effect of spinal blocks but can also be very severe if the anaesthetist giving an epidural accidentally punctures the membrane inside the spinal column. What happens in this case is that some of the cerebrospinal fluid leaks out and there is a drop in the pressure inside the skull, causing a very severe headache. The headache can be corrected with a blood patch: some of the woman's own blood is injected into the spine where it clots and forms a patch preventing any more fluid from leaking out. The headache usually goes within half an hour; without treatment it could last a few days or even a week. A headache can also be a sign of a womb infection, so it's always important to report one to your midwife.

> Ann had a Caesarean with her second baby: 'The thing that struck me most when I came round was the pain. I took every painkiller on offer and they did help. People say you've had major abdominal surgery, but I really didn't see it like that until afterwards. It also took some time for visitors to realize that I wasn't just going to get up and walk away from this. The major problems were sitting up, lifting, walking and getting into a good feeding position. You have to ask for help all the time. When you're in the special side ward for Caesarean mothers the midwives know that when you press the buzzer for help you mean business. But I was moved into

Your body after the birth

the main ward after a day and then I was treated just like anyone else. You have to be persistent.'

Rachel came home five days after her baby was born by Caesarean. Prompt action by her midwife and GP prevented an infection taking hold: *'It was the day after I came home that the pain really started to become unbearable. I was taking paracetamol. I told the midwife who suggested I soak in the bath. So we tried the next day and I got stuck on my hands and knees – the pain was excruciating and I simply couldn't move. Eventually my husband got me out and called the midwife who called the GP. Although there was nothing to see on the scar, the GP took a swab, prescribed some antibiotics and a stronger painkiller and got the midwife to rush the swab to the lab. It turned out I did have an infection and the scar started weeping a bit the next day. I took the antibiotics for ten days and the infection cleared up but I felt very stiff and uncomfortable for quite a long time.'*

Part Two

MOVING ON

When the midwife stops visiting you at home after ten days you may be left thinking that everything should be 'back to normal' now; if not at that point, then at least at your postnatal check-up which normally takes place six to eight weeks after your baby is born. But what if you don't feel 'back to normal'? One thing's for certain, you're not on your own, as you'll discover from some of the women who've contributed their experiences to this part of the book.

It is strange that after about seven months of regular clinic visits to check you are well *your* health suddenly no longer seems an issue – only that of the baby. But some of the problems associated with childbirth don't really emerge until later, and many women put up with a lot of discomfort because they think that's just the way it is after having children. But is it?

The following chapters describe some of the problems women sometimes experience and some of the possible solutions. In fact, there's often a great deal you can do to change things – although you may need a lot of determination. Most of the physical changes brought about by pregnancy and childbirth are reversible and there's rarely a case for putting up with things.

4
Getting back to normal?

'It took me three months to get my shape back but a year to feel physically well.'

Pregnancy is an incredible thing. The more you think about it, the more you wonder how your body can adapt to make room for another life and provide all the food to achieve such astonishing growth before the baby is born. Normally, your body's immune system would reject this kind of 'invasion' but – far from doing that – during pregnancy your body goes out of its way to change so that your developing baby is well fed and protected. If you appreciate the scale of these changes it can help you to understand why it sometimes takes a while for your body to recover.

How did my body change during pregnancy?

While you are pregnant you have:

- 6 litres (10½ pints) more water (some of it in the blood)
- 1.25 litres (2¼ pints) more blood
- enlarged kidneys
- fat deposits totalling on average 3.5 kg (7.5 lb)

Getting back to normal?

- up to fifty or even 100 times more progesterone hormone which relaxes all smooth muscle and ligaments, including the ligaments supporting your back

Added to this:

- Your heart beats faster and pumps more blood with each beat.
- Your heart may increase in size and is moved upwards and to the left.
- Your ribs flare out.
- Your womb gets eighty times bigger.
- You produce more melanin, which means your skin gets more tanned, freckly or otherwise marked.
- Your skin stretches over your breasts, abdomen and thighs.
- The joints in your pelvis soften and become loose.
- The duct system in your breasts develops.

Amazingly, experts believe that most of these changes are reversed within the first six weeks after your baby is born. So, for example, the amount of blood in your body returns to normal after forty-eight hours and your heart can stop pumping at such a rate because there is no placenta to feed with blood. The most dramatic reversals happen to your womb and cervix (see below) but not everything gets back to normal so quickly, as the following chapters illustrate.

The womb

As you know only too well, your womb (uterus) has to expand massively during pregnancy as your baby grows. The question is, how soon does it go back afterwards? In fact, it shrinks very quickly: in weight terms it's down from a high of 900g (2lb) at the end of pregnancy to just 100g (3½oz) after six weeks (compared to 60g (2oz) before pregnancy). But it never quite gets back to its pre-pregnant size – it'll be about 4cm (1½in) thick instead of 2.5cm (1in). So far as your shape is concerned, though, this is irrelevant. By the time your baby is ten days old the midwife probably won't be able to feel your womb above the pelvic bone any more. Unfortunately, any remaining bump that you can see is caused by slack or over-stretched abdominal muscles and the extra weight you're carrying (see Chapter 6).

The cervix and vagina

If you had a vaginal birth, your cervix which formed a 10cm (4in) wide circle for your baby to come through closes up almost entirely after one to three days. Your vagina has also been stretched considerably but doesn't completely regain its tone and tightness. This is particularly the case if there were any tears in the walls of the vagina during delivery. These tears heal very easily but tend to leave behind some non-elastic scar tissue. You may also find the entrance to your vagina gapes slightly. Although this sounds a bit alarming, it needn't matter if you have, or can develop, strong pelvic floor muscles (see Chapter 5).

Postnatal check

You'll be given an appointment for a postnatal check when your baby is six to eight weeks old. The appointment may be with your GP or at the local hospital. If you're offered one and you'd prefer the other, then ask.

Getting back to normal?

The postnatal check usually includes:

- taking a urine sample
- taking blood pressure
- an external examination to check your womb has shrunk back and possibly an internal examination to check the strength of your pelvic floor muscles
- contraceptive advice
- general discussion about how you are feeling
- possibly a cervical smear, especially if one was due during the time you were pregnant

If you feel you haven't recovered physically or emotionally from the birth, this is your chance to mention it and get your GP to help. Make a list of the points you want to raise if you think you might forget once you're at the surgery. If you aren't satisfied with the response you get, you could try another GP in the practice, ask your health visitor if she can help, or even contact your midwife for advice.

In many GP practices your postnatal check takes place at the same time as your baby's six- or eight-week check. This is obviously convenient – you only need to go to the surgery once – but it has the disadvantage that neither you nor the doctor are focused solely on your health and wellbeing. One way round this is to get your partner or a friend to look after the baby in the waiting room while your check is being done.

Q&A

I had a difficult delivery and I'm concerned the same thing might happen again if we wanted another baby. Can the doctor do any tests to see if I'm able to give birth normally?

It's not uncommon for women to feel let down by their bodies if they have a difficult labour – particularly if an assisted delivery with forceps or a Caesarean was required. It's easy for women to think they will never be able to deliver a baby normally, particularly if they hear people talking about the baby getting stuck or there being cephalopelvic disproportion (CPD) – a mismatch between the size of the baby's head and the size of the mother's pelvis. Normally, if the hospital staff suspect there might be a problem like this they will invite you back for a scan of your pelvis. This can show if it is small or an unusual shape but will rarely tell if you can deliver your next baby vaginally. That's because all the ligaments around your pelvis relax during pregnancy, increasing its size considerably. What's more, if you give birth in an upright position you get up to 28 per cent extra space – another 1cm (½in) across and 2cm (¾in) from front to back. And who's to say what size your next baby's head will be?

If you have any doubts at all about the way your labour went or you just want reassurance, you can contact the hospital direct or through your GP, to arrange a time to talk it through with the consultant.

I just don't feel things are the same inside any more. Will it ever be the same again?

It may not be until several weeks after the birth and after several times having sex that you start to wonder if you will ever feel the same as you did. Some women find sex very

Getting back to normal?

painful at this time, others feel their vagina is very loose, while others find they just don't have the muscles to squeeze their partner in quite the same way as before. It's right to say these things take time, but if you have any doubts at all about the way things have gone back together, it's really important to see your doctor for reassurance. That's easier said than done, of course: many of us find it difficult to talk about something so personal as sex, particularly unfulfilling sex, to our GPs! But there may be lots that can be done to help, so be bold: doctors have usually heard it all before and will be impressed by your honesty. If you're told everything is normal – even after a thorough examination – you may be able to get further help from a physiotherapist. See Chapters 5 and 9 for more details on specific problems and solutions.

Checklist: do you feel all right?

Use this checklist around the time of your postnatal check (after three months if you've had a Caesarean) to see how well you're recovering and whether there are any points you'd like to discuss with your doctor. Not everyone will answer yes to every question – we're all different and our experience of giving birth is different, but if something goes on being a problem it's worth getting help now, before you start accepting it as a necessary part of your new life.

- Can you sit comfortably?
- Can you walk a mile without getting backache?

Your body after the birth

- Can you climb the stairs or walk briskly round the block without getting out of breath?
- Can you jump up and down five times without leaking urine?
- Are you enjoying sex with your partner?
- Are you eating a healthy, balanced diet?
- Are you enjoying life?

Caroline says it took her a long time to get back to normal after giving birth to her daughter Lucy: *'It took much longer than I thought it would. I was still sore down below after three months and it turned out I had an infection which wasn't picked up – I suppose I didn't know any different and nobody checks after your postnatal check. I eventually had antibiotics when Lucy was about four months and by the time she was five months everything was fine.'*

5
Pelvic floor

Your pelvic floor is a multi-layered sling of muscles connected at the front and the back to the bones at the bottom of your pelvis (see below). Its job is to support your womb, bladder and rectum. There are three openings in the sling for the urethra, the vagina and the anus (see below). You use your pelvic floor every time you go to the toilet and when you make love. You also exercise it involuntarily every time you cough, sneeze or laugh suddenly. And that's where some of the problems start.

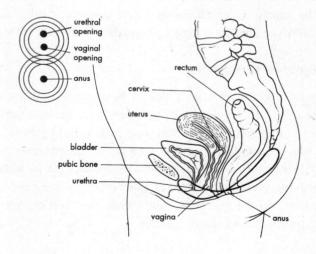

Stress incontinence

Incontinence means involuntary leaking or urine of even of faeces. Stress incontinence is the term used to describe urine leaking when you laugh, cough, sneeze or jump up and down. Stress incontinence is common in women whether they've had a baby or not, but especially if they have. In a study of 1,000 mothers, almost one in five said they were suffering some stress incontinence three months after their babies were born. More than one in ten were still suffering three years later. If you ask around among your friends you may find the problem is actually even more common than that. It's really not surprising when you think about it: during labour the pelvic floor has to cope with the weight of the baby and the pressure of contractions and one of its openings has to stretch to allow the baby through. It's also possible that some of the nerves supplying the muscle could be damaged during labour. Nerve damage is more likely if you were pushing for a long time in labour or needed forceps.

Getting back to normal

The good news is that your pelvic floor should get back to normal if you do regular exercises (see opposite) and particularly if you exercised it while you were pregnant. In general, the fitter you were before you had your baby, the stronger your pelvic floor muscles will be. Regular exercise such as walking and swimming will help alongside specific pelvic floor exercises. If you don't do the exercises, your pelvic floor will get weaker each time you have a baby vaginally.

Pelvic floor

Beating incontinence

- Do pelvic floor exercises daily (see box).
- Lose weight if you are overweight (to reduce pressure on your pelvic floor). If you're 5kg (12½lb) overweight it's like carrying a housebrick round on your pelvic floor!
- Take up walking or swimming.
- See a physiotherapist if things don't improve.
- Try using vaginal cones (see page 52).

Pelvic floor exercises

There are two basic types of exercise – slow and fast – to strengthen the muscles involved in maintaining tone and giving extra strength when you cough or sneeze. To locate the right muscles, imagine you are trying to stop yourself going to the toilet: you should be able to feel the muscles at the front lifting. Now tighten the muscles around your anus – your back passage – as well. That's your pelvic floor. If you're not sure you've found the muscles, try again, sitting on a hard chair, kneeling on all-fours or kneeling with your chest towards the floor.

Slow exercise: Lift and hold

Squeeze your pelvic floor muscles, lift and hold for as long as you can – until the muscles tremble – then release. Aim to hold for five seconds (you may need to build up to this).
  Repeat the hold five times.

Fast exercise: Twitch

Squeeze and lift your pelvic floor muscles in one twitching movement and release.
Repeat five times.

Ideally you should aim to do ten sets of these slow and fast exercises throughout the day, every day, for the rest of your life. In practice there will be days when you forget but you can find ways of making the exercises part of your routine. So you could do a set each time you brush your teeth, boil the kettle, change a nappy and pick up your baby. Don't leave the exercises until the evening – your muscles will be more tired then and the results could be discouraging.

If you find it hard to exercise your pelvic floor standing up, try kneeling on all-fours or lying down with your feet propped up on a low stool. Keep your knees slightly apart.

Prolapse

Prolapse means to slip forward or down out of place. A prolapse in one of the pelvic organs is caused by weak pelvic floor muscles and overstretched ligaments. A prolapse can mean that the bladder or womb is sagging into the vagina or the back of the vagina is sagging into the rectum. The most common type of prolapse after childbirth is the bladder sagging into the vagina. This causes a dragging sensation and you may be able to feel the protrusion – called a cystocele – like a soft grape if you insert a finger into your vagina. It's thought that about one in five women have some sensation of prolapse between fifteen and twenty-four months after giving birth. So prolapse is very common and the chances are that someone you know has one.

If you think you have a prolapse, see your GP who will refer you to a gynaecologist or a physiotherapist. The treatment often involves using vaginal cones (see page 52) or electrical stimulation to get the muscles to contract, and a physiotherapist may be able to loan you the equipment to use at home. But you will need to persevere with your own pelvic floor exercises as well. Don't give up: although it's unlikely the prolapse will be completely corrected, strong pelvic floor muscles should get rid of aching, dragging and incontinence.

In the worst cases it is possible to have a ring inserted to support a prolapsed uterus, or to have the prolapse repaired in an operation. But doctors are reluctant to operate on younger women or women who may want more children.

Checklist: do you have weak pelvic floor muscles or a prolapse?

Do you have:

- a dragging sensation around the vagina?
- difficulty keeping tampons in?
- stress incontinence (peeing when you sneeze or cough)?
- a need to go to the toilet frequently?
- fanny farts (see Chapter 9)?

Vaginal cones

These are small plastic cones into which you put tiny weights. You wear the cone in your vagina twice a day for fifteen minutes and gradually, over time, increase the number of weights inside. The theory is that your pelvic floor muscles will instinctively grasp the cone and so be exercised while you walk around and carry on as normal. Research seems to support their use. Cones and weights are available without a prescription but can be costly (£19.95 inc. vat and p&p for a set*), and not all women get on well with them. The physiotherapy department of your local hospital may have a stock of cones and a set of weights to give out on loan.

Faecal incontinence

If you've ever had severe diarrhoea and rushed to the toilet too late you'll have an inkling of how embarrassing and distressing faecal incontinence is for the few women who suffer from it. It's likely that this kind of incontinence is sometimes caused by nerve damage in the pelvic floor during the pushing stage of labour, particularly if forceps were used. The problem normally resolves itself after a couple of months but research has shown that three years after giving birth, around three out of 100 mothers are still suffering from faecal incontinence.

If faecal incontinence starts months or even years after giving birth, weak abdominal muscles and persistent constipation could be the cause. The sooner you get help from a physiotherapist the better. Pelvic floor exercises are vitally important and, even if you are doing your exercises regularly, it is important to get the physiotherapist to check that you are exercising the right muscles. The physiotherapist may also use a battery-operated device to stimulate and strengthen the muscles around the anus.

Very rarely, faecal incontinence is caused by a rectovaginal fistula – an internal opening between the bowel and the vagina, so that faeces appear to come from the vagina. This might happen if you tore very badly during labour and weren't stitched correctly. Don't let any embarrassment you feel about this stop you going to your GP and getting help as soon as possible.

Q&A

How do I know I'm doing my pelvic floor exercises right?
The most important thing is that you are exercising the right group of muscles. You can check this by squeezing the muscles while you are passing urine – you should find that you stop mid-flow. Make sure you empty your bladder properly after you've done this. You can do this test once a week to check your muscles are getting stronger as you exercise them regularly. Another check is to squeeze the muscles when you are making love: your partner should be able to feel what you are doing. Once you've got the right set of muscles you need to check that you are breathing normally while you hold, and that your abdominal muscles are relaxed.

I don't leak at all – why should I bother with pelvic floor exercises?
Because it will improve your sex life and stop you getting leaky when the muscles get weaker at the menopause, and because you don't know when the leaking might start (see below).

I had my last child over a year ago, so why has the leaking only just started?
Is it possible that you have stopped exercising your pelvic floor muscles over the past six months or so, perhaps because you weren't having any problems with incontinence? Unfortunately, pelvic floor exercises are for life: any postnatal gains in muscle tone will be lost if you stop exercising. Some people also think that if the nerves serving the pelvic floor were damaged during labour, this could lead to a gradual loss of tone in the muscles, with incontinence as a result. Even so, you should be able to strengthen the muscles with regular exercises (see box on page 49), and nerve damage may correct itself, so don't give up. If you want professional advice, ask your GP to refer you to a physiotherapist who specializes in incontinence.

There's no way I could talk about incontinence and prolapse with my doctor: I'd rather suffer in silence.
Lots of women feel like this and being embarrassed is quite normal. But being incontinent is miserable. It can stop you doing the things you enjoy like exercising and going out, and it can leave you feeling very bad about yourself. In the end it can make you depressed and possibly resentful towards your partner and your children. If you can't face talking to your doctor about it, think about making an appointment to see a private physiotherapist, buy your own vaginal cones and start doing pelvic floor exercises in earnest. You could also contact the Continence Foundation* for advice.

How soon can I expect to see results from pelvic floor exercises?
It's hard to give a straight answer to this since it depends on the strength of your pelvic floor at the moment. In general,

though, if you do ten sets of exercises every day you should feel an improvement within weeks rather than months.

Amy found she needed something to go wrong before she found the motivation to do pelvic floor exercises: *'It was about a year after I had Rory that I had a bad cough and I noticed I was leaking quite a bit. Even when the cough got better I kept thinking I was going to leak and after a couple of weeks I went to see my doctor. She got me an appointment with the gynaecologist who examined me and said I had a small prolapse. I was then referred to the physiotherapist who checked I knew how to do pelvic floor exercises and then lent me a set of vaginal cones for two months. I've read in magazines about women who rave about these cones but I didn't really like using them, although they did force me to think about doing pelvic floor exercises and things really did improve as a result. The physiotherapist tried to persuade me to buy my own set of cones and weights but I didn't. I'm okay at the moment, but I think if things got bad again I might buy them. At least now I know what to do.'*

Mary has two children aged four and two: *'I had good births both times, although I was pushing for over two hours the first time. It wasn't until my youngest was nearly two that I started having problems with stress incontinence – mostly when I was exercising. I found I needed to go to the toilet more often and urgently, and I had this dragging sensation down below. It also felt wrong down there, as though something had slipped. Things really improved when I started doing pelvic floor exercises and everything got better – no more wetting myself or having to go all the time.'*

6
Weight and shape

> '*I had a shower about an hour after he was born and I remember looking down and gasping out loud. My stomach was like one of those wrinkly old balloons you find behind the sofa two weeks after a party – all saggy and soggy.*'

Regaining their figure and losing the weight they put on during pregnancy are two of the biggest causes of complaint women have when their babies are four to six months old. By then, mothers have established some routines, got to grips with basic babycare and have a bit more time to think about themselves. Many women are also starting to think about returning to work at this stage and, having spent months in comfy casual clothes, are horrified to find that none of their work skirts fit at the waist. So are we expecting too much? Can you expect to get back to normal in terms of weight and shape? And if so, HOW and WHEN?

Weight gain in pregnancy

There are huge variations in the amount of weight women gain when they are pregnant: it could be anything from about 10kg

(1½ stone) to about 25 kg (4 stone). The average weight gain is around 12 kg (just under 2 stone). The variations can be caused by all sorts of factors (see chart, page 58).

Big weight gains

These could be due to:

- pre-pregnancy dieting keeping pre-pregnancy weight abnormally low
- taking less exercise during pregnancy
- overeating in pregnancy ('eating for two')
- conditions such as polyhydramnios (excess amniotic fluid)
- multiple pregnancy

Small weight gains

These could be due to:

- being overweight before pregnancy and living off reserves rather than gaining more
- being more careful about diet during pregnancy and eating fewer fatty foods

If you gained 12–13 kg (2 stone) or less, you may find you lose all but 4 kg (10 lb) or so within a few weeks of your baby being born. This remaining 4 kg (10 lb) represents your fat stores and the weight gain in your breasts. It will take time to lose this extra weight, but you can do it with a combination of sensible dieting and exercise for specific muscles, and the guidelines in this chapter should help. Some women seem to manage it instantly; for others it takes a year or more, depending on lifestyle, pre-pregnancy weight, basic metabolism and motivation. But even if your weight gets back to normal don't be surprised if you aren't exactly the same shape you were before.

Your body after the birth

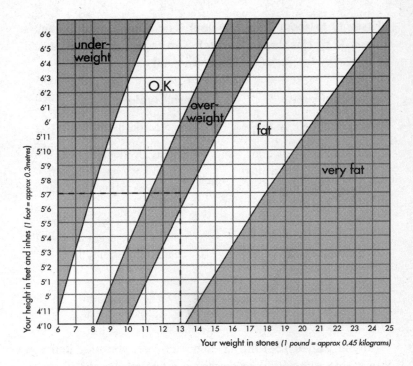

Are you the right weight for your height?

Changing shape

Many women find that having a baby changes their body, although in many cases the changes are more obvious after a second baby.

Weight and shape

- Your breasts may lose their elasticity and sag or droop. You may be told this is because of breastfeeding, but in fact it's caused by the hormonal changes in pregnancy and the time immediately following the birth. If you've always worn a good supporting bra you may notice the changes less. Breasts aren't made of muscle, so exercise won't change their shape. On the other hand, you can build up your pectorals – the band of muscles across the chest that give your breasts support. This may be particularly useful if you have very large breasts. Swimming breaststroke will help, and you can try the weights exercises 1 and 2 (pages 68–9).
- Your ribcage expands slightly towards the end of pregnancy to make room for your womb. Women who are slender may notice that this change isn't reversed after the baby is born: many tend to have a more square shape than before. If you wear loose tops, this may make no difference to you and you may be completely unaware of it. If you're trying to fit back into very close-fitting or shaped dresses you may find it a problem.
- Your abdominal muscles are stretched. This is rather like stating the obvious, but sometimes we need reminding what we've been through. If your abdominal muscles were weak before you got pregnant, it will take much longer for them to tone up, and longer still after a second, third or fourth pregnancy. That's not to say it can't be done, but it will take time and effort (see below and exercise 3, page 69).

A new image

Your changing shape presents you with a new image of yourself. If you were happy with yourself before you had your baby, you may find it hard to come to terms with this new image or you may even reject it and find yourself feeling resentful towards your partner and your baby – the people who 'made it happen'. These feelings can be made worse if the people around you refuse to see the problem. Work colleagues who got used to seeing a plump-faced pregnant woman may find it hard to remember what you were like before and refuse to acknowledge what is for you a very real problem. On the other hand, you may be under pressure from your partner to get back to normal. But what is normal? Actually, for some women it's perfectly normal to be a bit more curvy and cuddly and a bit less pert after having a baby. But that doesn't mean you can't tone your muscles – you can!

Checklist: What's your problem?

If you're unhappy about the way you look, use this checklist to work out what's really bugging you. Read through the questions once without your pencil, then go back to the beginning and think hard about each question before answering. Score each answer 0, 1, 2 or 3: 0 = not at all unhappy; 1 = slightly unhappy; 2 = quite unhappy; 3 = very unhappy.

How unhappy are you about:

- your weight?
- the image you project to others?
- the clothes you wear?

Weight and shape

- your hairstyle?
- your skin?
- your stomach?
- your breasts?
- your partner's reaction to you?
- your new role in life?
- your sex life?

For each question you've scored with a 3, look at the chart below and tick the things you could do to help yourself. Once you feel you've started tackling these areas you could run through the checklist again to see how your feelings have changed and to work out your new priority areas.

Weight	Check whether you are in fact overweight (see chart, page 58)
	Diet (see page 63).
	Join a slimming group such as Weight Watchers.*
	Join an exercise class.
	Go swimming on your own once a week.
Image to others	Ask two or three friends to be honest about how they see you.
Clothes	Buy something new and different – a new colour, a new style or something smart rather than casual.
	Go shopping with or get advice from a friend whose clothes you admire.
	Experiment with accessories – scarves, jewellery, belts.

Your body after the birth

	Organize a colour analysis evening (to find out what colours suit your complexion), for you and your friends.
Hair	Change hairdresser – ask around your friends for recommendations.
	Make a hair appointment and spend time discussing a new style and possibly a new colour.
Skin	Invest in a good moisturizer and use it day and night.
	Visit the Body Shop and ask for a free makeover.
	Explore ideas for getting more sleep (see page 123).
Stomach	Abdominal exercises (3, 4, 5, 6) (see pages 69–74) every day.
	Go swimming once a week.
	Go to an aerobics class once a week.
	Walk briskly for at least twenty minutes every other day.
Breasts	Pectoral exercises 1 and 2 (see pages 68–9) every day.
	Have a quality bra fitted at a department store.
	Check your posture (see page 92).
Partner's reaction	Talk to each other (you may be imagining things): be honest about how you feel.
New role	Work out exactly what you'd like to change.
	Talk to your partner to see if you can make changes at home.

Weight and shape

Sex life	Talk to other women about how they've adapted to motherhood. Talk to your partner. Read Chapter 9. Go to counselling together (for example, with Relate*).

Diet and dieting

Being overweight isn't good for anyone. It puts a strain on your back and your knees and it makes your heart work harder too. But there is a difference between obesity and wanting to lose a few pounds. You can use the chart (diagram 3, page 58) to see whether you are in fact overweight and by how much. Even if you are overweight, it's not a good idea to go on a strict diet if you're breastfeeding. In fact, if you are breastfeeding you'll be burning off an extra 500 calories a day anyway.

- Start by keeping a note of what you eat and drink each day for a week.
- Use different-coloured highlighters or felt tip pens to show up all the high-calorie, sugary and fatty snacks like biscuits, chocolate, sweets, crisps and cake (red foods), the fruit and veg (green foods) and the complex carbohydrates like bread, pasta, rice and potatoes (orange foods).
- The following week, aim to replace at least half the red foods with green or orange ones and repeat the diary to check what you've done. This will improve the nutritional content of what you eat without making you feel too deprived or hungry.

When you've stopped breastfeeding, if you feel you want to go on a calorie-controlled diet, consider joining a slimming group such as Weight Watchers.* These groups don't suit everyone but they can help with your motivation and keep you going during weak moments. When you're dieting you should aim to cut out most of the red foods, leaving two or three treats each week. You don't need to follow a complicated diet – smaller portions of your usual food served on smaller plates is often the best way (see Diet tips box). If you want to lose weight for ever you should aim to shed up to 1kg (1–2lb) a week. Anything more dramatic is unlikely to stay off.

Diet tips

- Use reduced-fat versions of dairy products such as cheese and yogurt.
- Use skimmed or semi-skimmed milk instead of full-fat milk.
- Use low-fat spread on bread or – better still – buy really fresh bread that doesn't need any spread.
- Trim fat off meat. Choose chicken (without skin) or fish rather than red meat if possible.
- Grill rather than fry your food, and let excess fat drain off.
- Choose tinned foods with no added sugar or salt (baked beans, kidney beans, sweetcorn, peaches, etc).
- Use wholemeal versions of bread, flour, rice and pasta.

Weight and shape

Exercise

If you exercised regularly during pregnancy, you will probably find it easier to carry on after your baby is born – not least because many antenatal swimming and aerobics classes also cater for postnatal women as well. If, on the other hand, there wasn't the time or opportunity for exercise during pregnancy and you've been concentrating all your energies on the baby, you may find you're at a loss where to begin. Don't panic! You can find those muscles again, lose weight and rebuild your stamina, strength and suppleness. But it will require effort and patience. No one can do exercise for you and there's no instant formula. Exercise works gradually and you'll feel and see its benefits gradually if you stick with it.

Some private fitness clubs and NHS obstetric physiotherapists run postnatal exercise groups in some areas. The great thing about these groups is that you can take along people you have met in antenatal classes who are at roughly the same stage as you, and you can be part of a supportive group of friends who all understand how difficult it is to shed that last stone or half-stone along with the three extra inches and the floppy paunch. If you haven't seen any classes advertised ask your midwife or health visitor. Don't join a general keep-fit or aerobics class until your baby is at least twelve weeks old. Leave it longer if you have any joint problems or you're suffering from stress incontinence. Always tell the instructor you have had a baby and opt out of any exercise you find uncomfortable. Stop if you feel dizzy.

If you don't want to join an exercise class or go swimming –

perhaps because these activities are too 'public' for you at the moment – you can easily devise your own exercise programme to lose weight, tone your muscles and regain your confidence. Although again, you'll need to be determined.

- Once your baby is eight weeks old you can aim to go for a brisk walk at least every other day. Your walk should last at least twenty minutes and should leave you puffing. If you're not puffing, your heart isn't getting enough exercise and you won't be burning off many calories. As you walk, tighten your abdominal muscles every few seconds for extra benefit. This kind of exercise is easy to incorporate into most lifestyles: if you're at home you can do it while pushing the pram. If you're at work you can use part of your lunch break to walk.
- Get hold of an exercise video or book specially designed for women who have had babies.* Watch or read it all the way through twice to get a feel for the exercises described, try them out, and then work out what you could do every day or every other day at a set time. It may help to make a pact with a friend about this. If you agree on the same programme you can compare notes and motivate each other even though you are exercising in private. Home exercise doesn't need to involve complicated routines: marching, arm swinging, side bends, knee lifts and simple stretches will make up a good programme. But be careful to follow all safety instructions about warming up and protecting your back as you exercise, and stop immediately if you feel dizzy or sick.

If you're only concerned with toning up flabby abdominal muscles – in other words 'getting rid of your stomach' – the best exercise is to do curl-ups (exercises 3, 4 and 5 below). These are a modified form of sit-ups – modified to make them

Weight and shape

safe. Never do full sit-ups or straight-leg sit-ups: you will put a tremendous strain on your back. When you exercise your abdominal muscles regularly you:

- shorten muscle fibres which have been stretched
- strengthen muscles which have been weakened
- close any separation in the muscles (see page 82).

Don't do any strong abdominal exercise until a midwife has checked your abdominal muscles (see Chapter 7).

Exercise for the first six weeks

It's a good idea to start gentle exercises as soon as you can after your baby is born, but don't overdo it in the first six weeks and remember to get your midwife to check you over before you do any curl-ups. (If you've had a Caesarean, see Chapter 3 for advice on exercise in the first six weeks.) Try the following:

- Ankle circles – in both directions, while you are lying down. Repeat whenever you think of it!
- Foot pedalling – bending your feet towards you and stretching them away while you are lying down. Again, repeat whenever you can.
- Pelvic floor exercises – as many as you can (see page 49).
- Pelvic tilting – see below (exercise 3). Repeat three times a day.
- Leg sliding – start with a pelvic tilt, then, while your abdominal muscles are pulled in, slide one leg slowly

down the bed or floor until you feel your back start to arch, then pull it back. Repeat a couple of times. As time goes on you should be able to get the leg out flat. Remember to keep your back pressed down. Repeat three times a day.
- Basic curl-ups – see below (exercise 4). Repeat three times a day.

Exercise 1: for pectorals (breast support)

- Lie on your back, knees bent, feet flat on the floor and pushing your lower back into the floor.
- Hold a 500g–1.5kg (1–3lb) weight in each hand (a large can of baked beans will do if necessary) and put your arms out from your sides so you make a T shape with your body.
- As you breathe out, keep your arms straight and bring your hands together above your chest.
- Breathe in as you lower your arms slowly to the ground. Repeat ten times.

Exercise 2: for pectorals

- Lie on your back as for exercise 1, with the same weights in each hand.
- Put your hands on your chest, breathe out and push the weights up towards the ceiling.

Weight and shape

- Hold for one second and bring the weights down slowly as you breathe in. Repeat ten times.

Exercise 3: for abdominals

Pelvic tilting)

- Lie flat on the floor with knees bent and together, feet flat.
- Put your hand behind your back in the gap left by your curved spine.

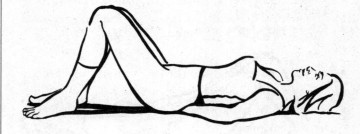

- As you breathe out, pull in your abdominal muscles and try to press your lower back into the floor. Hold for a count of four and release. Repeat eight times, building up to twelve times.
- As your muscles get stronger you should be able to hold for longer but stop if your muscles start to tremble.

Exercise 4: for abdominals

Curl-ups

- Lie on your back with your knees bent and feet flat on the floor.
- Place your hands on the tops of your thighs.
- As you breathe out, pull in your abdominal muscles, press your lower back to the floor, tuck your chin in towards your chest and lift your neck and shoulders as far off the floor as you can, sliding your hands towards your knees as you curl up.
- Hold for a count of four, then uncurl back to your starting position.
- Repeat eight times, working up to fifteen times.

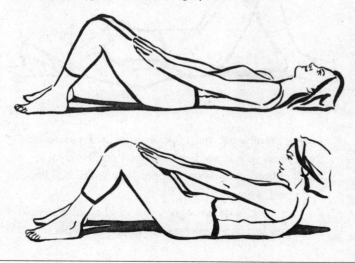

Exercise 5: for abdominals

Advanced curl-ups

- Don't do these until you can comfortably do sets of fifteen ordinary curl-ups and your baby is six weeks old.
- Cross your hands over your chest (each hand on the opposite shoulder) and repeat curl-up as above. Repeat eight times, working up to fifteen times.

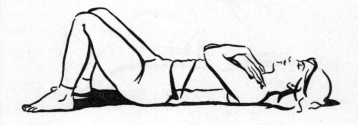

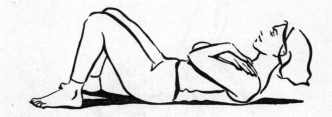

Exercise 5: (continued)

- When you can do this comfortably, you can make the exercise even stronger by putting your hands beside your ears, bringing your bent knees towards your chest and then straightening your legs slightly as you curl up. Repeat eight times, working up to fifteen times.

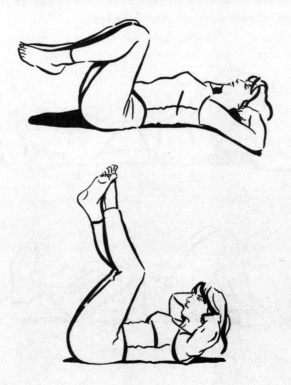

Weight and shape

Exercise 6: for abdominals

Angry cat

- Get on all-fours on the floor, with your back flat, your knees under your hips and your hands under your shoulders.
- As you breathe out, pull in your abdominal muscles and arch your back. Hold briefly, then release.
- Return to a flat-back position and repeat eight times, working up to fifteen times.

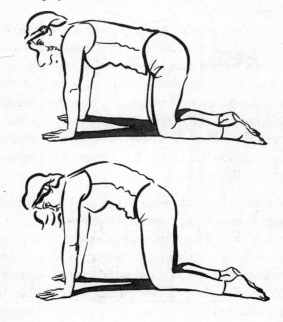

> When you've finished exercising it's a good idea to stretch your muscles as they cool down. Hug your knees to your chest for a count of ten and then stretch right out on the floor for a further count of ten.

Q&A

I was told in antenatal classes that breastfeeding helps you get your figure back but my midwife said it makes you retain fat. Which is true?
Breastfeeding in the early days helps your womb to shrink back more quickly but in the longer term it varies from woman to woman. Some women find that breastfeeding uses up the fat reserves they laid down during pregnancy and that they suddenly shed the extra weight between three and six months after the baby is born. Other women find they don't lose the weight until they stop feeding. Whichever way, breastfeeding doesn't affect your muscle tone, which is often the problem with regaining your figure.

I hate the way my breasts look now – they're all droopy like an old woman's. Is there anything I can do about them?
Unfortunately there's very little any of us can do to change the shape of our breasts. However, the exercises for pectorals (see page 68, exercises 1 and 2), along with breaststroke swimming, may help develop the muscles which support your breasts. Wearing a really classy bra that gives you good support and improves your contours can make you feel good about yourself,

Weight and shape

so if you can afford to splash out on some new underwear, go for it. But even that may not be enough if you feel depressed every time you get undressed or have a bath. Talking to your partner about the way you feel and getting his reassurance that he still loves the way you look may help. Talking to other women who've had babies can also reassure you that you're not alone in feeling like this and may even make you laugh at the situation.

I have absolutely no willpower when it comes to dieting and I find being at home means I'm in the fridge or the biscuit tin the whole time. What can I do to lose weight?

Being at home surrounded by food (and being responsible for preparing a lot of it in many cases) makes it extremely difficult to keep to any kind of diet. The best advice is to keep it simple, to think about a combination of diet and exercise, and not to be too hard on yourself. Big resolutions ('I'll never eat crisps, sweets, cakes or biscuits ever again') are often broken in the first twenty-four hours. Take one meal at a time. So, for example, at breakfast-time, stop putting jam on your toast, or leave off the butter and use a reduced-sugar jam; switch to skimmed milk on your cereal and use sweetener rather than sugar in tea or coffee. Prepare snacks of raw carrot, celery and cucumber in advance for weak moments and buy a variety of fruits for your fruit bowl rather than a mega-pack of crisps. Don't forget you are probably burning off a lot of energy looking after your baby – particularly if you walk rather than drive the car everywhere. Aim to walk for at least twenty minutes most days. Some people find it helps to make a pact with friends: agreeing not to offer each other biscuits and cake when you meet for coffee is a good starting point!

How soon can I start exercising?
There are certain exercises you can – and ideally should – do in the first week of your baby's life, others which you can add in after your midwife has checked your abdominal muscles (see page 82) and more after you've had your six-or eight-week check. The advice is different if you have had a Caesarean section (see page 32).

When can I start going swimming again?
As soon as your perineum has healed and you have stopped bleeding: before that there is a risk of infection. Bleeding normally stops after a few weeks (see page 4).

> Polly found it wasn't until after she had her second child that she had problems with her weight: *I didn't put on much weight in either pregnancy and it was quite easy to lose it straightaway, but I think I slowed down mentally after I had my second baby and lost all my willpower. It was something to do with being at home more and I always seemed to be making food for someone and then finishing it up to save throwing it away. Plus I had no time to exercise, so I put on a lot of weight. I made a couple of attempts at doing aerobics in the evenings but in the end I had to make it a priority and pay for someone to look after the children while I went to a gym two or three times a week. I feel much better for it – both physically and mentally.'*
>
> Fiona, a mother of two children aged four and two, comments: *'You tend to make new friends after you've had your*

Weight and shape

first baby and they don't know what you looked like before. So in one sense it doesn't matter what you look like: they don't realize how much you've changed, although you still know it yourself. The question is, can you accept it?'

Andrea believes her concerns about weight in the past were caused by her lack of confidence in herself: *'I was worried about my weight after I had my second baby but I think it was all part of my low self-esteem. I'd always been overweight as a child and then I lost weight when I was in the sixth form and it completely changed me – I had so much more confidence. When I couldn't shift the weight after being pregnant I felt somehow I was going back to the way I was as a teenager. I had no willpower to diet and I was just too tired. Having no time to exercise is still a major problem. Exercise changes my attitude to food: if I feel fit I don't eat cake. But as time has gone on I've come to terms with my new shape. I wear baggier, less fitted clothes, and so what if I don't look really slim? I know my husband loves me no matter what.'*

Louise found she lost all the weight she'd gained in pregnancy very quickly – especially after her second child was born: *'I've always had to watch my weight since I was a child but over the past ten years or so I've managed to stay fairly slim. The thing I noticed after having Andrew, though, was how flabby my stomach was. It took me a while to realize that dieting wasn't going to shift it, so I started going to aerobics and it really has helped. I enjoyed getting out on my own as well.'*

Julie, a mother of two, says: *'The thing I found hardest to cope with was the way my breasts drooped after I stopped* breastfeeding my second baby. They were never very big but now they seem ridiculous. I think I went through a stage of thinking I just wasn't very womanly any more. Fortunately my partner is very caring. When I told him how I felt he was very reassuring and convinced me it didn't matter to him, which helped a lot.'

7
Backache

Your back is an amazingly complex piece of engineering and there's huge potential for things to go wrong with it. Backache is a warning sign and should never be ignored. You can take painkillers like aspirin, ibuprofen or paracetamol, but that doesn't deal with a problem which could get worse and lead to long-term damage. Backache during and after pregnancy is very common, but that doesn't mean it has a single cause or a single treatment, or that it should be accepted as 'just one of those things'. If you have a regular backache, it's important to get help. If your GP won't take you seriously, you could consider going to an osteopath or a chiropractor (see page 96).

Pregnancy, childbirth and backache

It takes up to six months for your softened ligaments and other connective tissues to get back to normal after pregnancy, as levels of the hormone relaxin drop. Since your back is supported by these ligaments (along with your stretched abdominal muscles), women with newborn babies are very vulnerable to backache. Whether there is a direct connection between events during labour and the onset of backache is another matter.

Checklist: Where's the pain (see opposite)

Backache is a catch-all term which covers a wide range of problems, each with slightly different solutions. So the first thing is to work out where you feel the pain. Is it in your

- neck and upper back? (cervical region)
- mid back or between your shoulder blades? (thoracic region)
- lower back? (lumbar region)
- buttocks? (sacral region)
- coccyx or 'tail bone'? (coccygeal region)

Back problems can also cause pain elsewhere in the body if a nerve in the spine is being irritated. Do you have pain in your

- legs? (possibly a problem in the lumbar or sacral region)
- arms? (could be a problem in the cervical or thoracic region)
- buttocks, groin, hips or knees? (may be a problem in the thoracic or lumbar region)

Birth engineering

If your baby was born vaginally, she had to find her way through a curve in your pelvis – rather like putting your foot in a wellington boot. To help her, your pelvic bones, including the bones in your lower spine, moved and got out of her way, with the help of your soft and stretchy ligaments. It's not surprising, then, if many women have some backache after even a straightforward labour as their joints settle back into position. If your labour was prolonged for some reason – perhaps because the baby was in an awkward position or had a large head – your joints may have had to move more and so may take longer to recover.

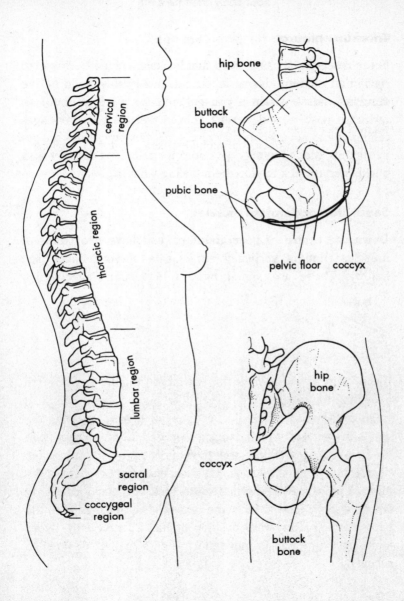

After an epidural

Some research has suggested that backache could be linked to having an epidural during labour. In theory this could be the result of muscle strain if you got into (or were put into) an awkward position and weren't able to feel the pain messages telling you to move. This may also apply to women who are put in stirrups (the 'lithotomy' position) for a forceps delivery with a local nerve block to stop them feeling what is going on.

Separated abdominal muscles

Down the centre of your abdomen you have two bands of muscles running vertically either side of your navel (see below). These are joined by a thin fibrous layer which

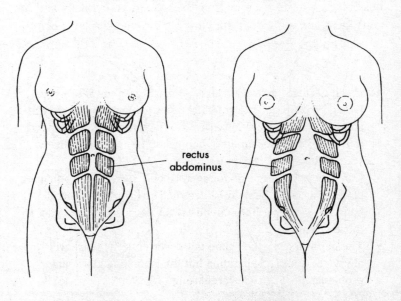

rectus abdominus

Backache

stretches during pregnancy, allowing the muscle bands (called rectus abdominus) to separate slightly. This separation – normally only an inch or two – should close up within a week of your baby being born. If your baby was very large, or you had twins (or more!), or you have a very narrow pelvis and were 'all out front' during your pregnancy, it's possible the bands may have separated further. At worst the separation could be 12.5–20 cm/5–8 in wide and run from your ribs to your pelvis. Because your abdominal muscles are so important in supporting your back, this kind of split can lead to terrible backache.

If you are slim it may be possible to see the gap between your rectus abdominus under the skin as two bulging ridges, and many women can feel it as a 'hole'. To check for separation before you exercise, lie on your bed, bend your knees and lift your head and shoulders up. Now feel around the level of your tummy button. Move your fingers from side to side until you feel the two bands of muscles.

- If you have severe backache it is very important to see your GP and a physiotherapist before you do any postnatal exercise: some exercises could make the gap bigger and you will need to take special precautions, such as crossing your hands over your abdomen when you exercise.
- Consider using some abdominal support such as body-shaping underwear or a double thickness of Tubigrip (a support bandage, available from chemists) for extra support as you move around.
- The gap will close over time but never entirely: there will always be a slight separation but this shouldn't cause any problems if the muscles are strong.

Your body after the birth

Jill's back problems didn't really start until her second son, James, was about six weeks old: *'I'd been very anaemic, but once I felt fit again I think I just did too much and didn't think about my tummy muscles although I'd been told they'd split and that I'd need extra help. Even two months after James was born I could put my fingers through my tummy. It was awful – like jelly. I saw the physio who gave me stomach exercises which I did every day but my back got worse. It was painful whenever I moved and I couldn't walk upright. In fact, I could barely walk at all sometimes. I saw a rheumatologist who told me I needed cortisone injections into my spine, but I didn't want that so I just put up with it. I was lucky I didn't have to do any housework or gardening. When I went back to work I had to have a special chair, carry a cushion round with me and use a suitcase on wheels for taking files home! Going to London on the train was agony. It was over two years before I felt better. I still do specific exercises for my back, and although I can't swim very far or do weights I have recently started playing squash again, so I must be getting better.'*

Julie is six feet tall and thinks her backache is made worse by her height: *'I have a bad back anyway as a result of a horse riding accident when I was younger, but it doesn't help having a heavy baby and being tall. I've learnt that I really need to bend my knees a lot and concentrate whenever I pick up Emily. I have to make sure I'm always looking at her, not picking her up on my side. You can do it, but you do need to be aware of your back all the time.'*

Weak abdominal muscles

Women with weak abdominal muscles or women who were bed-bound for long periods of time during pregnancy are also likely to feel the after-effects in terms of backache. Ideally, anyone in this position should have the chance to see a physiotherapist soon after the baby is born to get help with specific strengthening exercises which can be done safely.

Stress and tiredness

One of the major causes of backache among women with three-, four- or five-month-old babies is fatigue – that lethal combination of stress and tiredness that affects your mood, your energy levels, your posture, your motivation to exercise and your attention to detail. So you no longer sit properly to feed your baby, you forget to bend at the hip before picking her up, you slump in a chair for the evening, you fall asleep feeding while propped up against the headboard of the bed (which doesn't support your head) and you walk around with drooping shoulders which tense up every time your baby cries. That's what prolonged lack of sleep does to you, and it's easy to see how it can cause problems by straining the muscles which support your back. If you think this could apply to you, ask yourself these questions:

- Do my health and comfort matter?
- Am I unhappy like this?
- Would I like to feel energetic again?

Women often neglect their own health and well-being after they have a baby and, after a few months, it's very easy to feel

Your body after the birth

there's no solution to your problems and that you just have to soldier on the best you can, especially if you're on your own, your partner works long hours or you have no friends or relatives living locally. But it doesn't have to be like this. See page 123 for ideas for combating tiredness and recouping your 'sleep debt' – all those hours you're owed. So far as backache caused by tension is concerned...

- Exercise – go to a swimming or aerobics class where there is a crèche for babies (or take turns with a friend looking after each other's babies). Far from using up the little bit of energy you've got, exercise makes you feel more energetic, helps you sleep better when you do get the chance, and makes you feel more positive by producing endorphins (your body's natural painkillers). If you do aerobics, tell the teacher about your backache so she can check that you are exercising properly and not straining yourself.
- Use essential oils such as lavender, marjoram and clary sage in the bath or in a burner to help you relax. Chapter 12 (page 141) has more details about these essential oils and general warnings about using them.
- Read the sections below on posture and protecting your back, and the advice on positions for feeding (under Thoracic backache) and have a go for one day to start with. Even if your backache doesn't improve instantly you may be surprised how good it makes you feel about yourself when you stand tall and sit well.

Severe back pain

Very rarely, women suffer from osteoporosis brought on by pregnancy. This can lead to broken bones towards the end of pregnancy or such severe constant back pain afterwards that doctors discover an undiagnosed fracture in the spine. The good news is that with a combination of good diet and exercise most women in this situation find they recover well and their bones get back to normal. To find out more about osteoporosis contact the National Osteoporosis Society.*

Self-help for backache

NB: If you have severe backache or a pain which lasts for more than a few days you must see your GP.

Cervical backache

This kind of neck, shoulder and upper back pain is common if you are very tense, have been sitting with your head unsupported or are hunched against the cold.

- Massage around the neck and shoulders can do wonders for backache caused by muscle tension. Using carefully chosen aromatherapy oils can also help as they can lift your mood and help you to relax (see page 141).

Your body after the birth

- Change chairs or use extra cushions to give your neck and head more support.

Thoracic backache

One of the most likely causes of pain in the mid back is an uncomfortable or awkward position for feeding the baby. This applies whether you are bottle- or breastfeeding. In both cases you are usually in one position for some time and if it's the wrong position you could be putting a strain on your back.

- Sit to the back of the chair or against the back of your bed so that your back is supported and that you aren't hunched or slumped backwards. Don't perch on the side of the bed. If you're sitting, your feet should be flat on the floor. If the chair is too high, rest your feet on a couple of telephone directories. It may also help to put the baby on a cushion as you feed (see diagrams opposite). Once you get home, ask a breastfeeding counsellor* to visit you and advise about sitting and positioning for feeding.
- Try massage to ease the pain. A full body massage given by a trained aromatherapist, for example, can be wonderfully soothing and can free up a lot of the tension which is causing your pain. But it's not difficult to learn simple massage strokes, and a massage given by someone you love (and who loves you) can be just as good if not better.
- Learn how to relax. If you were shown how to breathe calmly and deeply in antenatal classes, carry on practising this whenever you have the chance to sit or lie down for five minutes. Imagine all the tension disappearing from your body as you slowly breathe out. Do a mental check on every part of your body to make sure you are not tensing and that all your

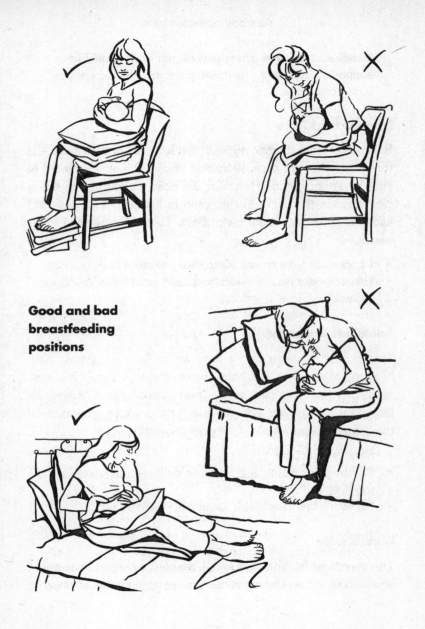

Good and bad breastfeeding positions

muscles are relaxed. Every part of your body should be supported, including your head and arms. Playing relaxing music can help.

Lumbar backache

Backache in the lumbar region – the low part of your back – is the most common area of trouble and may not be related to your pregnancy at all. However, the extra weight of pregnancy can increase the curve in the spine in this area (see page 81) and can make you stand awkwardly. This can make the joints unstable.

- Check your posture and make sure you are lifting correctly.
- Use hot-water bottles, warm baths and gentle massage to ease the pain.

Sacroiliac backache

This is a common place to have backache after giving birth because of the way the baby moves through the pelvis (see above). If you have pain at the front of your pelvis as well it's important to see your GP: you may have a slight separation of the symphysis pubis joint (see page 99). Otherwise:

- Soak in a hot bath.
- Try the pelvic tilting and angry cat strengthening exercises on pages 69 and 73.
- Lie with a hot-water bottle against the painful area.

Coccyx pain

The coccyx or tail bone is a small, triangular-shaped bone at the base of the spine. During labour the coccyx moves backwards to make more space for the baby to come down. Although this isn't painful at the time it can be very sore afterwards and can make it very uncomfortable to sit down.

- Sit on a Valley Cushion (see page 13 for hire details).
- If you are breastfeeding, ask a counsellor to help you find a good position for feeding lying down.
- Use ice packs or hot packs or a TENS machine (which provides electrical pulses to block pain signals) to ease the pain (Boots the Chemists hire out TENS machines or the physiotherapy department at your local hospital may be able to lend you one).
- Take anti-inflammatory painkillers such as ibuprofen.
- Ultrasound treatment from a physiotherapist or an osteopath may also help: ask your GP to refer you.
- Corticosteroid injections may help if the ligaments are inflamed.

Unfortunately there are no quick and easy solutions for a bruised or inflamed coccyx, but keep trying different options. Not being able to sit comfortably isn't funny and it can ruin the precious time you have with your baby.

> Tricia found her coccyx was incredibly painful after the birth of her second child: 'To start with I didn't realize the pain was coming from the coccyx: I thought it was the episiotomy and general soreness in that area. But when the episiotomy got better I realized the pain was more localized around the coccyx and going up into my lower back. The worst thing was not being able to sit normally. I had to sit on one buttock all the time, and getting up to run after my three-year-old was agony. I tried using a Valley Cushion but I didn't find that helpful. My GP suggested steroid injections but I didn't

fancy that, so I saw an osteopath who manipulated my lower back, used ultrasound and did stretching with the palm of her hand on either side. She couldn't press directly on to the coccyx because that was too painful. After each treatment I was in agony but it did get slightly better over time. Even so, three and a half months on it was still painful and I had to sit on one side in a soft chair, so I made an appointment to have the injections. I thought they'd be really painful but they weren't, and they really worked.'

Good posture

- Stand tall.
- Keep your shoulders down.
- Lift your ribcage.
- Balance your weight on both feet.
- Don't lock your knees.
- Pull in your tummy.
- Tuck your bottom in.

Protect your back

- Make sure pram handles are at the right height for you: you shouldn't have to stoop or hunch your shoulders.
- Feed in a comfortable position (see above).
- Change and dress your baby on a high surface – just below elbow height is ideal. If you want to do it on the floor, half-kneel or sit upright with your baby between your legs (see diagrams opposite).
- Put your baby bath on a table or use one which fits across the bath. NEVER attempt to lift a baby bath when it is full of water. Fill it with buckets of water and either empty it in the

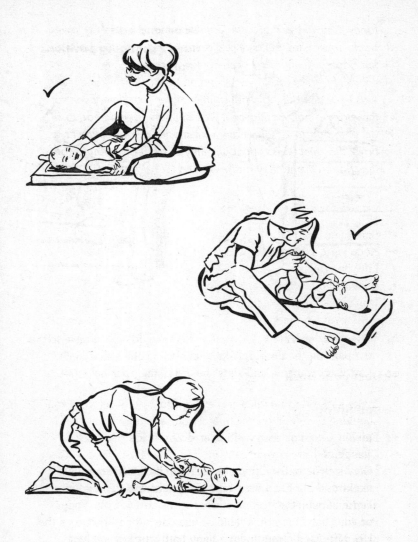

Good and bad nappy changing positions (floor)

Your body after the birth

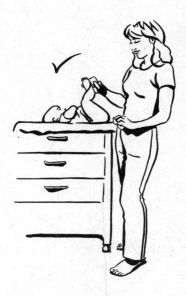
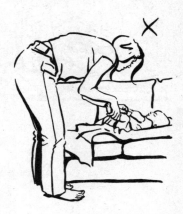

Good and bad nappy changing positions (standing)

same way or leave it for someone else to do. If you have to put the bath on the floor, half-kneeling will protect your back.
- Lower the cot side and squat before lifting your baby out.

Good lifting

- Ideally, avoid all heavy lifting or divide loads (e.g. wet washing).
- Get as close to the thing you're lifting as possible, put your feet around it, bend your hips and knees and get a good grip. Don't lift with outstretched arms – this strains your upper back.
- Keep the load close to your chest and your knees apart.
- Use your leg muscles to lift, not your abdominals.

Backache

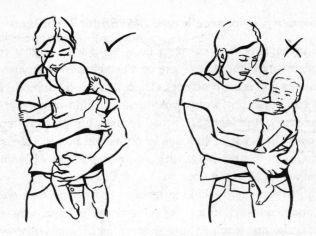

Good and bad carrying positions

Later on . . .

- Sitting, crawling and toddling babies need a lot of lifting and carrying. Use the same lifting technique described above. Whenever possible avoid carrying your baby on your hip (see below): give her a cuddle instead.

Exercises for back pain

Although these exercises are very simple to do at home by yourself it makes sense to see your GP first to discuss your backache and to get his or her advice about exercising. Alternatively, you could go to a local postnatal exercise class if there is one in your area (see page 65). If you prefer to exercise at home, use the pelvic tilting and angry cat exercises on pages 69 and 73 to strengthen your back.

Osteopathy, chiropractic and Alexander Technique

Both osteopathy and chiropractic – so-called 'alternative' or 'complementary' therapies – are now established as mainstream treatments for back problems. There are slight differences in the techniques, but both involve manipulation to correct misalignments in the joints. In broad terms, chiropractors tend to use more thrusting techniques to reposition bones; osteopaths tend to do more stretching and gentle repositioning of ligaments around a joint to free it up.

The Alexander Technique teaches correct posture so that your body can work in a more relaxed and efficient way. Alexander Technique teachers* use gentle manipulation and exercise to help you retrain your body's posture and movements, to reduce the stresses and strains which are causing backache.

Q&A

Are baby slings a good idea? Can they cause backache or make it worse?
A sling is much better than hip-carrying but it can cause a strain on your back if the baby isn't held close to your body. If possible, experiment with different slings until you find one that feels comfortable. Remember to check your posture when you're using it: tuck your bottom in, drop your shoulders and lift your ribcage.

I started having backache about a year after my baby was born. Could there be a connection?
It's possible that all the lifting and carrying involved in looking after a baby or toddler is starting to tell – particularly if your

Backache

child is heavy. Make sure you protect your back when you lift (see page 94). If the pain goes on or gets worse, see your GP, especially if you have other symptoms such as stress incontinence or pain inside your pelvis. It's possible you may have a prolapse – where the womb slips forward into the vagina (see page 50) – or fibroids (benign tumours). These can both cause pain in the lower back.

My doctor says I have a trapped nerve in my back. What does that mean?
Your spine is made up of bony vertebrae layered with discs made of a jelly-like substance. These discs can bulge out of place and press on one of the nerves coming out of the spinal column. If this happens you'll feel the pain shooting down your arm or leg probably – wherever the nerve leads. Sometimes a pinched nerve can cause pins and needles rather than pain. One of the most common forms of the problem is sciatica where a disc in the lower back presses on the sciatic nerve and the pain runs down one leg to the foot. Bed rest may help. The protruding disc normally shrinks back into place after a while. Most people with sciatica find it goes within three months, but three months is a long time if you've got a new baby to look after. Ask your GP if he or she will refer you to an osteopath.

8
Other joints, aches and pains

Unless you were previously doing a job involving a lot of lifting, walking and carrying, your lifestyle has probably changed significantly since you had your baby. Looking after a baby is very physical and even if you've returned to work, you're almost certainly doing more physically than you were before. All the lifting, carrying, bending and just holding involved in caring for a baby is bound to put your body under considerable strain at times. It's not just your back but your knees, shoulders, calves and arms which may ache and develop niggly pains.

Chapter 7 contains tips for protecting your joints when you lift and carry, and for reducing the stress and tension which cause so many aches and pains. If following these pointers doesn't help, and your aches and pains keep coming back every day for a week or so, it's worth going to your GP in case something else is causing the problem. Some women are affected by the hormonal disturbance in pregnancy to the extent that they get joint problems. But these should be resolved once your hormones have settled down. It's possible you may have a calcium deficiency which can cause muscular aches and pains (see Q&A below).

Alison has suffered badly with joint problems since her son Marlo was born seven months ago: *'I had a skiing accident*

Other joints, aches and pains

ten years ago when I tore the ligaments in one knee, and now, since having Marlo the same knee has been swelling up. The doctors think the weight of the baby brought back the old problems and now it's very painful to walk. I've been having ultrasound treatment from the physiotherapist every week but it doesn't completely clear it. It's a pain inside – apparently it's the soft palate on the knee which swells. It's not terrible – just annoying. It means I can't do any aerobic exercise and I can't walk very far. They haven't said how quickly it will get better. I've also got painful finger joints which are a bit of a mystery. First thing in the morning when I try to move them they're really painful. My GP thinks it might be because of excess fluid in my body because I'm still breastfeeding, but she's really not sure. And I'm also having ultrasound treatment for my shoulder which I threw out when I was carrying Marlo's car seat. There's no mystery about that – he weighs 22 lb!'

Lorraine also had shoulder pain within a couple of months of having baby Carrie: *'The pain was in my shoulder and upper back and was obviously something to do with the joints being soft and all the lifting I was doing. I had three sessions with the physiotherapist using ultrasound treatment and me keeping packs of frozen peas on it. It got better, although very occasionally I still feel it as a burning pain so it's obviously left some kind of weakness.'*

Symphysis pubis dysfunction

The joint at the front of your pelvis – the symphysis pubis – is actually a pad of cartilage (like the cartilage in your nose) which links your hip bones. While you are pregnant the ligaments which hold this pad in place soften because of the high levels of the hormone progesterone – sometimes to the extent that the joint opens up creating a gap – a condition called symphysis pubis dysfunction (SPD). In some severe cases the ligaments can separate completely from the joint: this is known as dyastasis symphysis pubis. Both conditions can be incredibly painful and disabling: some women have great difficulty walking or are actually wheelchair-bound as a result. Climbing stairs and turning over in bed can be almost impossible. But in many cases the condition resolves after the baby is born and progesterone has gone back to normal or near-normal levels. For some women, however, the problem doesn't resolve quickly. For others, it only emerges during labour or even a few weeks after the baby is born.

The pain is felt very low down over the joint, in the groin, the hips and sometimes down the inner thighs. If you suspect you may have this problem, your GP can refer you for an x-ray. It's possible the x-ray won't show a great deal of separation at the joint as some cases are caused by swelling rather than separation, but the treatment is still the same.

Treatments for SPD include:

- anti-inflammatory painkillers
- support from a belt or Tubigrip elastic bandage
- using a TENS (Transcutaneous Electronic Nerve Stimulation) machine for the pain
- bed rest
- avoiding standing and movements which separate the knees
- walking with small steps and with the help of crutches or a frame

It is vital to see a physiotherapist for advice on all aspects of treatment and for help with a gradual exercise programme which will strengthen the joint. It's possible that osteopathy or chiropractic (see page 96) may help, but choose a practitioner who has experience of dealing with SPD.

Unfortunately there are no guarantees the problem will resolve quickly. It can take weeks, months or even years in the most extreme cases. Some women find that the pain is worse in the second half of their menstrual cycle, because of an increase in progesterone, the ligament-relaxing hormone.

If none of the above treatments work and the separation is very severe, it is possible to have an operation to fuse the joint. If you've had SPD once it's likely to happen again in your next pregnancy, so if you do get pregnant again, make sure you tell your midwife and see a physiotherapist early on. Information and support are available from the British DSP Support Group.*

Hip pain

Very rarely, women develop osteoporosis of the hip during pregnancy and this may not be discovered until after the baby is born, perhaps even a couple of months afterwards, although the pain is likely to be constant and severe. Osteoporosis is a condition in which bones become so fragile they can break very easily. No one is quite sure why pregnancy causes osteoporosis in some women but the outlook is very good: even in severe cases it seems the bone loss may be reversible. For more information about osteoporosis contact the National Osteoporosis Society.*

Headaches

A lot of women find they suffer from headaches or even migraines after they have a baby. In some cases there is a direct link to childbirth: if you have an epidural, for example, there is a one in 100 chance you could have a 'dural tap' where the epidural needle punctures the membrane inside the spinal column, with the result that some of the cerebrospinal fluid leaks out and reduces the pressure inside your skull. This isn't dangerous but it can cause a very severe headache which may last up to a week. The headache will feel better if you lie flat, drink plenty of fluids and take paracetamol for two days while the hole heals itself. If this doesn't work or the headache is very bad, it can be corrected with what's called a blood patch: some of your own blood is injected into the spinal column to seal the puncture.

In many other cases, however, there is no obvious and direct link between childbirth and the start of headaches except that now you have a baby to look after and that can be stressful and tiring. Many headaches are caused by tension, stress and sleep deprivation (see page 122). Others can be put down to the progestogen-only mini Pill which you may be taking now for the first time in your life since it is compatible with breastfeeding (see page 115).

One of the problems with headaches is that we can keep taking the tablets and hope they will eventually go. But headaches caused by stress often don't respond to painkillers. In fact, there's evidence to suggest that some recurring and persistent headaches are actually caused by overusing painkillers! In any case, the manufacturers of paracetamol, aspirin and ibuprofen recommend you see a doctor after two or three days if your

Other joints, aches and pains

headache doesn't get better. It's obviously worth getting checked out but, unless you have very severe symptoms or there is something obviously wrong, the GP probably can't do very much at this stage.

That doesn't mean you just have to live with the misery of repeated headaches. It may help to keep a diary which you can take to show your GP if the headaches don't stop. A simple calendar chart in which you record the type of headache (sharp, dull ache, throbbing, etc.) and other symptoms (nausea, vomiting, visual disturbances, etc.) along with details of your period (if periods have returned) may reveal a pattern. Many women find they have headaches in the two weeks before their periods start because of hormonal changes. The doctor may also want to know:

- how long the headaches last
- whether they come at a certain time of day

It may also help if you can make time for relaxation – in a hot bath, for example, with some carefully chosen aromatherapy oils (see page 141). You could also try massaging the temples.

Q&A

I had horrible varicose veins during all three of my pregnancies. They seemed to go after the first two but this time I've still got them after three months. Are they likely to go?
Varicose veins normally disappear after your baby is born but women who've had several babies and whose veins are badly varicosed may find they never recover completely. If your varicose veins only appeared during pregnancy and you've regained

your normal weight, there's no reason to think you'll get any more. If you are really distressed by the ones you have, an operation to remove them is relatively simple, but there are often long waiting lists for treatment on the NHS. In general, you can help prevent varicose veins getting worse by exercising and wearing support tights which are virtually indistinguishable from ordinary stockings and tights these days. You may be able to get these on prescription.

My wrist and fingers have started to go numb, tingly and painful. Sometimes I can hardly lift my baby because of it. What's causing this?
It's possible that you have carpal tunnel syndrome, a condition in which swelling presses on one of the main nerves running through your wrist. Some women get carpal tunnel syndrome while they are pregnant and it usually resolves after the baby is born. But a few women do get it afterwards when it seems to be linked to breastfeeding, although no one knows why. Your GP can confirm whether you have got carpal tunnel syndrome. If so, it may help to have a wrist splint and take anti-inflammatory painkillers. In the meantime, rest your wrist as much as possible.

I've been told I have a calcium deficiency. Does that mean I will get osteoporosis?
No. As you obviously know, calcium is needed to build up your bones (your 'bone density') to protect them against the crumbling of brittle bone disease or osteoporosis. It's quite normal for bone density to drop during pregnancy and while you are breastfeeding because of the baby's demands for calcium. But studies have shown that, two years later, everything is back to normal. Only in very rare cases does pregnancy lead to osteo-

Other joints, aches and pains

porosis (see page 87). Calcium deficiency can cause muscular aches and pains and these should improve if you increase the amount of calcium in your diet. So, drink a whole pint of milk a day (skimmed milk actually has slightly more calcium than whole-fat milk) and make sure you get extra calcium in the form of yogurts, cheese, sardines, pilchards, dark green vegetables and dried fruit such as figs and apricots.

9
Sex

Some experts say women shouldn't have sex until at least three weeks after giving birth because there's a very small chance of complications. But, in reality, many women don't even think about sex until their babies are a few months old (see box below). Even if you had an elective Caesarean, sex may be difficult for the first six weeks or so because your abdomen will feel tender; orgasm may be painful for three months or more if it makes your uterus contract. The important thing is that you and your partner talk about the situation and are both comfortable with it.

Sexual statistics

- One in five couples start having sex within four weeks of delivery.
- One in ten couples wait until between five and seven months after the birth.
- Some couples haven't had sex even one or two years later.
- A year after childbirth, only half of all couples are having sex as often as they did before – for a variety of reasons, including tiredness, loss of libido and lack of privacy.

Getting started again

If you have a gap of several months in your sex life the biggest problem may be finding a way to get started again. You can avoid some of the physical problems if you:

- Feel your vagina yourself first to see if it hurts.
- Use KY jelly if your vagina is dry.
- Don't attempt to have penetrative sex unless you are fully aroused.
- Choose a time when there's a good chance the baby may stay asleep, and after a feed if you are breastfeeding, so there's less chance your breasts will leak during intercourse.

If the problem is emotional rather than physical, start by holding hands, snuggling up together while you watch TV, kissing and cuddling – and see where it all leads. This is the approach many sex therapists recommend as it helps a couple to rediscover each other. A Relate survey found that seven out of ten women lacking interest in sex or having arousal problems reported improvements after therapy.

A new relationship

Try not to be disappointed if your sex life isn't the same as it was before: having a baby does bring about changes for both of you. That doesn't mean your relationship is ruined – it's just different. Many couples say it's a question of quality not quantity: they have sex less often since they became parents but when they do make love it's much better, perhaps because they have a deeper caring and appreciation for each other.

One thing is for certain, though: sex should not be painful. If it is, you need help to find out why and what can be done to solve the problem.

Dryness

It's quite normal for your vagina to be dry for some time after your baby is born – it just takes a few weeks for the usual lubrication to come back. A dry vagina can become very sore during sex, particularly if you aren't aroused, so it makes sense to use a lubricating gel such as KY jelly.

Vaginismus

Vaginismus is a painful condition in which the muscles around the vagina go into spasm and shut so tight that sex is often impossible or, if not impossible, then extremely painful. It's an involuntary reflex reaction – not something which you can control. After childbirth vaginismus can be caused by memories of a difficult birth or it may be a response to the pain of an episiotomy or bad tear which is still healing. It can even be a flashback to sexual abuse in the past. It can also be the result of over-tight stitching. Vaginismus is difficult for you and your partner: he feels rejected and you feel doubly upset, because you love him but your body won't let you show it.

Although there are techniques for overcoming vaginismus, involving internal examinations and vaginal cones, the most important step for many women is speaking to a female sex therapist. This can bring any unconscious fears or anxieties out into the open. Learning how to relax is invaluable and the therapist can help you with this. Your GP may be able to refer you to a sex therapist, otherwise you can contact Relate* or the Association of Sexual and Marital Therapists.*

Restitching

Sometimes there is a longer-term problem with the way the perineum has been repaired or the way it has healed. If this is the case, your doctor might suggest you go back to hospital to be 'restitched' in a procedure called 'refashioning the perineum'. This is done under a local anaesthetic (see story below). Most women find the stitches heal more quickly and are less troublesome this time, not least because they aren't recovering from the birth at the same time.

Elizabeth found sex very painful after her baby was born: *'I had an episiotomy and lots of stitches and it was sore for a long time because of the scar tissue. Sex was impossible because I was just tensing up all the time. After about nine months I went to the doctor and he suggested I should be restitched. It was done in hospital under a local anaesthetic and took about an hour. The doctor also told me to concentrate on relaxing which really helped a lot.'*

Marion wonders whether she was stitched too tightly: *'There was no way we could have full sex for months after I had my baby. It was incredibly painful every time we tried and I always had to ask Dave to stop which meant he was really annoyed and I got really upset. But there was nothing I could do about it – I was in absolute agony. After about ten or twelve weeks I spoke to the nurse at the clinic and she said maybe I had been stitched too tightly, and when I saw the GP he said I could have it redone if I wanted. But I wasn't very keen and so we tried massaging the skin and eventually it was okay – whether the stitches loosened up or I was less tense I don't know, but things have been fine since.'*

Lorraine found a quick solution to her problem: *'The first time we tried to have sex it was about four weeks after Carrie was born and it was incredibly painful – I had to ask Peter to stop. I went to the GP as soon as I could and she found there were some loose stitches which had to be taken out. After that it was fine.'*

Perineal pain

It's hardly surprising that most women have some pain around the perineum – the skin between the vagina and the anus – after they give birth. After all, the skin has been stretched and put under a lot of pressure. If the skin has torn or been cut (in an episiotomy), again it's not surprising if it takes time to heal. But how long? One study found that on average it took a month for women to feel comfortable walking and sitting and three months for them to feel comfortable during sex. But for one in five women the healing process was longer – two months for general comfort and six months for sexual comfort. Having a forceps delivery tends to delay healing.

So what can you do to ease the discomfort and speed healing? And when should you get help?

- Persist with your pelvic floor exercises (see page 49): they may help with pain as well as incontinence.
- Take warm baths with added essential oils for relaxation and healing (lavender, geranium and rosemary are all supposed to be healing oils, but see page 142, for general warnings about using essential oils).
- Get help if you feel the pain or discomfort goes on for more than two months, especially if it is making you feel depressed.
- Ultrasound treatment and a similar technique using pulsed electromagnetic energy are sometimes used to help healing, although there is mixed evidence about their benefits. Even so, it may well help to spend some time with a physiotherapist talking about the problem and exploring options for treatment. Your GP can refer you to a physiotherapist, although there is often a waiting list, so don't delay.

Episiotomy healing

It generally takes longer for women to recover from an episiotomy than from a perineal tear. Sometimes the episiotomy can damage nerve endings, resulting in a particularly painful patch which you can't bear your partner to touch. Scar tissue can also cause pain during sex. One solution is to change your position during sex, to avoid the sore patch. Nerves which have been cut during an episiotomy should heal eventually, but in the meantime sex may only be possible if you use an anaesthetic gel or spray to numb the pain.

Pain inside the vagina

If you feel pain high up inside your vagina when your partner penetrates deeply then it's possible the ligaments around your cervix were torn during labour. These tears will heal but it makes sense to avoid deep penetration until then.

Vaginal pain can also be the result of a prolapse, where the bladder sags into the vagina (see page 50).

Loose vagina

The walls of the vagina are incredibly elastic and contract amazingly after you've had a baby. But the vagina doesn't completely regain its tone and tightness, with the result that it may feel slightly 'looser'. You may notice, for example, when you have a bath that your vagina fills with water – which comes out when you stand up! If the muscles around the vagina are weak you may also experience 'fanny farts' during sex or if you sit up suddenly, as the air in your vagina is expelled. Some women find this quite funny; others are upset, ashamed, embarrassed or even devastated at the change in their bodies.

If you had stitches after your baby was born, it's possible you were stitched too loosely, but this would only affect the entrance to the vagina and wouldn't account for the unfortunate noises or the vanishing bathwater. Improving muscle tone in your pelvic floor (see Chapter 5) may help during sex as you will be able to grip your partner's penis more tightly.

> Julie, mother of two, says: 'The first time we heard the fanny farts we were making love and we couldn't believe it. I had no idea why it was happening and assumed it was my "fault" for not having a nice tight vagina. It doesn't happen every time we have sex and it's not something I think about or worry about, but when it does happen I still feel shocked and a bit disgusted.'

Q&A

How soon after you've given birth can you start having sex again? Should we wait for the bleeding to stop?

Some doctors say it's best to wait three to six weeks before having sex, and in fact most couples wait at least a month. Whenever you choose to start again, your partner should be gentle and must be prepared to stop if you experience any pain.

We tried to have sex about four weeks after our baby was born but it was really painful and I've been too frightened to try again. What can I do?

If there was a physical problem at four weeks – a tear or bruise which was slow to heal, for example – it may well have cleared up by now. It may help if you examine yourself, perhaps when you are in the bath and feeling relaxed, so you can be confident you don't feel pain any more. If you still experience pain after a few months there are several possible reasons – an undissolved stitch, a piece of scar tissue, the after-effects of an episiotomy, infection or a trapped nerve ending, for example. If you've had stitches, it may be you've been stitched too tightly, leaving a narrowed entrance to your vagina. There are successful treatments for these problems, so do get help from your doctor.

I'm breastfeeding and every time we have sex I leak milk everywhere. The first time it was funny, now my partner gets annoyed and I feel really messy. What can we do?

The simple answer is to make love just after you've fed the baby. In reality, though, that may not be possible if your baby is difficult to settle. Understanding why leaking happens may help: basically the same hormone which releases the milk – oxytocin – is produced when you are sexually aroused. If your partner avoids putting any pressure on your breasts that may help delay any leaking, so try going on top.

Since giving birth I've completely lost my libido – I just never feel like making love. What's happened to me?
It's not unusual for a woman to find so much pleasure in handling her new baby that she doesn't feel the need for sex. It's also possible that the hormonal changes involved in breast-feeding can cause a temporary loss of libido (although some women have quite the opposite reaction). It's likely your sex drive will return in time, but if it doesn't you can get some simple but very effective help from a sex therapist.* A therapist can help you examine your feelings about yourself and your partner. It may be that you aren't happy with your body and that you have a poor self-image. If so, you may find some useful advice in Chapter 6. Or you may feel exhausted by motherhood and resentful of a partner who doesn't help very much. If so, it's hardly surprising your libido is low! The therapist can help you work through some possible solutions to these problems. On the other hand, if you feel you're very much in demand these days, you may just need some personal space: taking time out on your own one or two evenings a week might help.

It's a year after I had my baby and I'm still not enjoying sex – it isn't painful but it feels so different – do you think there is something wrong?
It's possible your pelvic floor muscles haven't got back to normal and if so, both you and your partner will notice a difference. You can strengthen your pelvic floor by tightening,

holding and releasing the muscles regularly throughout the day (see page 49). If you had stitches after your delivery, it's also possible you were stitched up loosely. If you think that's so, or you want reassurance that everything is normal, ask your doctor to give you an internal examination to check. On the other hand, your lack of enjoyment in sex could be linked to your emotions – there may be tensions in your relationship, for example, which mean you don't get fully aroused. If so, it may help to talk to a sex therapist.*

When is it okay to get pregnant again?
There's no absolute answer to this question. It partly depends on you, your physical recovery from the birth and the way you are feeling emotionally. It's partly a financial decision, perhaps related to return to work, your career and the maternity-leave options open to you. And it's partly a matter of personal preference: some women prefer the idea of having children close in age, others want to get potty training out of the way before having another baby. If you're asking what a doctor would recommend, again there's no absolute answer, but there is some evidence to suggest that both mothers and babies benefit physically and emotionally if there is a two- or three-year gap between children.

Contraception

Your priority with contraception is probably effectiveness! Few women are comfortable with the idea of getting pregnant again within weeks or months of giving birth. But this is also a time to review your choice of contraception, and your thoughts may have changed now you've had a baby. For one thing, if you are breastfeeding you won't be able to use the combined Pill because the oestrogen affects the quality and quantity of breastmilk. The progestogen-only mini Pill is suitable and extremely effective – if it is taken at the same time each day – as is the IUD (the coil), although this can't be inserted until your baby is at least six weeks old. But some women decide they've had enough tampering with their hormones and their bodies and want something else.

Diaphragms and condoms can be very effective if they are used properly. If you used a diaphragm before you were pregnant you will need to have a new one fitted because your shape will have changed as a result of the pregnancy. If you later lose a lot of weight (more than half a stone) it's best to check that your new diaphragm still fits well.

In the longer term, when your menstrual cycle has settled into its new pattern (see page 139), you may want to use natural family planning which involves monitoring the changes in your body which lead up to ovulation and avoiding sex (or using another type of contraception) on 'unsafe' days. You need to be taught this method, but if you're interested, a good starting point is the book *A Manual of Natural Family Planning* by Dr Anna M. Flynn and Melissa Brooks (George Allen & Unwin, 1988).

> Breastfeeding on demand is not a reliable contraceptive, although you may find your periods don't return until you stop feeding. Watching for that first period is no good either since you can ovulate – and get pregnant – before it comes.

10
Skin and hair

'Fantastic tan and freckles like you've never seen before!' That's how one woman recalls the way her skin changed during pregnancy. Such changes are very common because your body produces more of the pigment hormone melanin while you are pregnant. This is responsible for the appearance of new moles, dark patchy colouring on the face (called chloasma), the dark areola around the nipples and the linea nigra – the dark line running from belly button to pubic hair – as well as the easier tanning and freckles. Blonde women may also notice their hair gets darker or at least looks darker, particularly around the parting if they have one. Black women may notice their skin get darker or that pale patches develop on the face and neck.

Chloasma (and any pale patches) should start to fade as soon as your baby is born and should have gone completely within a couple of months. Other changes may be slower to reverse (such as the linea nigra) or may be permanent (such as new moles). If you get pregnant again, staying out of the sun will help to minimize all these skin colour changes.

Stretch marks

Unfortunately there's nothing you can do to prevent or treat stretch marks which were the result of your skin thinning to cover your bump, your breasts and any other parts of you that grew! When your baby is about six months old you'll probably find the stretch marks have faded to a silvery colour so they aren't quite so obvious.

Hair loss

It's bizarre, but while you are pregnant your hair gets locked into a growing phase and doesn't fall out (at least, nowhere near as much as normal). This has the wonderful side-effect of making your hair thick and glossy at a time when many women can do with a morale booster. Unfortunately the opposite happens when your baby is born and your hair gets locked into a resting phase during which there's no new hair growth and a lot of hair falls out. You may find you lose quite alarming quantities of hair for up to two years, but this is only the hair you would have lost in the nine months you were pregnant. Things will get back to normal eventually.

Q&A

Why have I suddenly got loads of spots? Most of my friends had spots while they were pregnant but my skin was great then.
Did you suffer from spots before you got pregnant? If so, it's possible that your body liked the extra hormones it had during pregnancy and they cleared up any tendency to acne which was there beforehand. And don't forget that your hormones are all

Skin and hair

over the place after you've given birth and it will take a while before they settle down and you can see what's normal for you now. If these spots don't clear after a couple of months, and you've finished breastfeeding, you might consider going on to the combined Pill to boost your oestrogen, although there are no guarantees: you may find it has the opposite effect and makes the spots worse. Probably the most effective non-prescription remedies you can buy for acne include an ingredient called benzoyl peroxide. You could also talk to your GP about the options, including antibiotic creams or tablets for severe acne.

Is there anything I can do to get rid of stretch marks?
Very little, unfortunately. It's possible that massaging vitamin E oil into the skin may encourage new skin cells to grow, and this may in turn help with scarring.

What could be causing the dark rings under my eyes?
This could just be tiredness or it's possible you are anaemic (see Chapter 11). Ask your doctor to do a blood test and, if necessary, prescribe an iron supplement. Check you are eating well: if you don't eat red meat, you need to make sure you get enough iron from non-meat sources, such as bran flakes, spinach, lentils, wholemeal bread and tinned tuna.

Why is my hair falling out in handfuls?
This is almost certainly due to the reversal of changes which occurred during pregnancy when your hair stopped falling out and grew much thicker (see above). This natural hair loss can go on for up to two years. If you're really worried, though, talk

Your body after the birth

to your GP. It's extremely unlikely, but very occasionally hair loss is caused by a permanent hormone imbalance.

> Jo enjoyed her deep tan during pregnancy but wasn't so impressed when, having finished breastfeeding, she found a line of tiny moles roughly along her bra line: *'I suppose they were there all the time but I was too big to see them! I was very freckly while I was pregnant and I think those skin changes have lasted, though it's hard to tell. I suppose it doesn't really bother me: I think you just have to accept that your body has changed. It's a bit like stretch marks – you don't like them but they're part of your life, and after a while you just stop noticing them. There's too much else to think about!'*

11
Tiredness

Tiredness is a fact of life for new parents. But having people tell you it comes with the territory doesn't help – it's still something you have to live with. Tiredness is especially common among women who have had a Caesarean, but anyone who's been through a long labour is bound to have missed out on one night's sleep, if not two. It has been described as the cruellest blow of nature, that just as you need sleep most you're faced with twenty-four-hour responsibility for a baby who may want cuddling, feeding and changing every thirty minutes or so. The first few days may pass in a blur of excitement as you find out about your baby, with the result that often the tiredness doesn't really hit until your partner has gone back to work and perhaps your friends and relatives are 'leaving you to get on with it'. Although tiredness is an obvious problem, unless you do something about it, the lack of quality sleep can lead to more subtle but serious problems.

Sleep deprivation

Sleep deprivation is a recognized problem among doctors (who all experience it to some extent during their training). Laboratory studies show that the effects of prolonged sleep deprivation are:

- mood changes and irritability
- hallucinations
- memory lapses
- speech difficulties

Studies of junior doctors have also shown that lack of sleep impairs creativity. In other words, although they could perform routine tasks they were unable to think laterally. For women at home looking after babies this is the equivalent of operating on automatic pilot, which isn't very nice in the long term. There's no doubt that having your sleep disturbed over and over again – however much you love your baby – can be very stressful and can cause tension headaches (see page 102).

What helps?

No one understands the agony of a sleepless night better than another new mother and it's amazing how much it helps to know someone else is suffering the same as you! (If all your friends have babies who sleep ten hours a night and nap three times during the day then it's time to make some new friends....) But talking is never going to be enough: you need to get more sleep and make the most of the sleep you do get.

Tiredness

Getting more sleep

- Set an alarm for 10pm at the latest and go to bed then, regardless.
- If your baby needs a late-evening breastfeed, express some milk and ask your partner to give it in a bottle so you get a longer stretch asleep.
- Sleep whenever your baby or toddler does: resist the urge to tidy up or cook the dinner during this time.
- For daytime naps put a note on the door asking people to call back, switch on the answerphone and unplug the phone in your bedroom.
- Stop trying to do too much (see box on page 126).

Tips for improving your sleep

- Have a warm bath before you go to bed. Add a couple of drops of lavender oil to the bathwater.
- Try a herbal sedative. Passiflora, hops, wild lettuce, valerian and skullcap are used in various over-the-counter preparations and are all mild sedatives.
- Only take drinks containing caffeine (these include tea as well as coffee) in the morning and early afternoon. Try fruit teas instead.
- Avoid alcohol in the evening – it can cause early-morning waking.
- Try to leave at least three hours between a meal and going to bed.
- Exercise during the day or early evening rather than later or you'll be too hyped up to sleep.

Despite a hectic life with a baby and toddler, Janet finds it difficult to get to sleep at night, but she has developed a successful night-time routine: *'I have a pair of headphones under my pillow with an old story tape that I know back to front. When I can't get to sleep I switch it on and I never hear the end! Even so, I rarely sleep all night – even when the baby does. But I reckon if I've had four or five hours solid then I'll survive! I don't want to get wound up about it – that will just increase the stress and make things worse.'*

Tiredness and depression

The link between tiredness and depression is complicated. Tiredness can be a symptom of depression but it could also be part of the cause of depression – if constant lack of sleep along with responsibility for the baby and lack of support is getting you down, for example. It's important to be honest with yourself as you try to work out the root of the problem (see Chapter 12).

Anaemia

The symptoms of anaemia are:

- tiredness
- breathlessness
- pale skin
- weakness
- fainting or dizzy spells

Anaemia is caused by a reduction in the amount of haemoglobin in the blood. Haemoglobin is the part of your red blood cells which enables them to carry oxygen to all your muscles. It's hardly surprising, then, that without enough haemoglobin you feel weak and tired. A simple blood test can confirm whether you are anaemic and whether you need iron supplements. In the meantime, make sure you get enough iron in your diet. If you don't eat red meat you can get iron from bran flakes, spinach, lentils, wholemeal bread and tinned tuna.

> Jill lost a lot of blood after her second son was born and it was suggested she should have a blood transfusion: 'But I said I didn't want one. I asked if I could get myself back to normal and they said, "We'll see." I felt very weak and had to stay in hospital for four days because I was so anaemic. I couldn't even walk across the ward to start with. Even when I came home I had to rest all the time: I couldn't do anything except look after the baby. They gave me iron supplements and I had a diet sheet which was wonderful – lots of chocolate! It took a long time to get back to normal. I had to take the iron for about two months. But I did it in the end.'

Thyroid problems

A few women suffer from an underactive thyroid (hypothyroidism) following childbirth. The symptoms of this are:

- exhaustion
- weight gain
- being short of breath
- constipation
- dry skin
- puffy ankles
- mood swings
- feeling cold all the time
- thin hair

Hypothyroidism can be corrected very easily with hormone tablets to replace the missing thyroid hormone, thyroxine.

> **Are you trying to do too much?**
>
> If you're trying to re-create the myth of superwoman then you're heading for trouble! Caring for a new baby is a full-time job – everything else has to take a back seat. So:
>
> - Make priorities.
> - Learn to say no to additional tasks.
> - Ask for and accept help – from parents or friends.
> - Work out times each week when you will do nothing but relax.
> - Do important jobs during your least tired times, if you have them!

Q&A

I can't believe I'm so shattered: I used to work twelve-hour days in a highly stressful job managing people and not feel as tired as this. Why do other people seem to cope much better?
Other people ALWAYS seem to cope much better! At least you are being honest about your feelings. Women who've had busy jobs where they are in charge sometimes find the unpredictability of life with a baby extremely difficult to handle. This kind of emotional stress can be very tiring. Don't forget, too, that you probably had uninterrupted sleep and leisure time to yourself before. If you can restore some of that – by keeping one evening

Tiredness

a week just for you or by insisting on a catch-up sleep every weekend – you may be able to restore some sense of control to your life. You may also find your tiredness eases as you get into a routine: try planning something each day (for example, shopping, meeting a friend, discussion group, exercise class, swimming, mother and baby group or clinic visit).

I know everyone feels tired with a new baby, but my baby's nearly eighteen months and I still feel shattered. Could there be anything else wrong with me?

It's possible you are anaemic or that you have an underactive thyroid. With both of these it's likely you'd have some other symptoms (see pages 124 and 125). Your GP can check for both conditions with a basic blood test. If you don't have any other symptoms it's still worth going to the GP, but spend some time first thinking about your lifestyle, the amount you try to cram in and the quality and quantity of the sleep you get.

Checklist

If you want to try to work out what's behind your tiredness or you're thinking about seeing your GP, it may help to think about these questions:

- Do you have a regular bedtime?
- How many hours of uninterrupted sleep do you get?
- Do you find it difficult to fall asleep?
- Do you wake (without reason) during the night and have trouble getting back to sleep?
- Would you say your tiredness was mostly mental or mostly physical?
- How long have you felt this way?

Your body after the birth

- Do you have any other physical symptoms?
- Is there a time of day when you feel least tired?

It took Louise a long time to realize how tiredness was affecting her: 'I think my son was about fifteen months old when I suddenly realized I was dragging myself around. I had no energy for anything, least of all looking after him. I went to the doctor and she was very sympathetic. She did some blood tests but they were all negative. I think she thought I was a bit depressed, and perhaps I was. Looking back, though, it's hardly surprising I was tired: I'd been commuting three hours a day since Jack was five months old, he was still getting up at night, and I was just exhausted. In the end I changed my job and went part-time and as he started to sleep more things got better. But I do wish I hadn't tried to do so much.'

12
What about my hormones?

As soon as the placenta detaches from the wall of the womb, your hormones start to go a bit haywire. While you were pregnant you had about fifty times as much oestrogen and progesterone as normal. Within hours of the birth the extra has virtually disappeared. At the same time your body starts producing large quantities of another hormone – prolactin – which is involved in milk production. Prolactin levels remain high for some time, regardless of whether or not you breastfeed, suppressing oestrogen and progesterone and boosting your endorphins, your body's natural painkillers. Your thyroid gland also responds to childbirth by producing less hormone than it did before you got pregnant. But what impact does this hormone roller-coaster have on your mood and emotional state?

> **Hormones**
>
> Hormones are the body's chemical messengers. They control all your body's functions including your growth, your sexuality, your fertility, the way you burn up food, and your response to stress. But your hormones – and the way you respond to them – are unique. According to a leading

> expert, it's one of the great unsolved mysteries of medicine why some women are more affected by their hormones than others.

Baby blues

The so-called baby blues which are very common on the third or fourth day after a baby is born may be caused by these dramatic changes in hormone levels. They may also be tied up with the loss of any initial euphoria or excitement over the baby and any physical discomfort you're feeling. The baby blues are also more common in first-time mothers, which suggests that there may be a link with lack of confidence in handling the baby and the responsibility of motherhood.

Baby blues and postnatal depression are not the same thing, although some people think that if the baby blues are not handled carefully they could lead to postnatal depression. But mild postnatal depression (see box below) may well be part of a perfectly normal adjustment to parenthood. That doesn't mean you shouldn't get help – in fact, it's possible that the women who don't get help are those who are more likely to slide into more severe postnatal depression. Your GP should organize a simple test to check you aren't suffering from an underactive thyroid or anaemia.

Baby blues vs postnatal depression

	Baby blues	*Mild postnatal depression*
Starts	day 3–7	any time up to a year afterwards
Lasts	1–3 days	months or years if untreated
Symptoms	weeping for no reason, mood swings	easily upset and irritated, hypersensitive
		no self-confidence
		no energy for anything
		unable to concentrate
		feel guilty and a failure
Treatment	encouragement, support, rest	encouragement, support, talking, practical help, time without the baby, professional counselling

Postnatal depression

Severe depression is an energy-sapping, personality-changing disorder that is not your fault. It doesn't mean you are an inadequate person or that you have failed in any way. It is not something over which you have any control. Experts disagree about what causes postnatal depression and the chances are it is not any one thing but that there are a variety of possible causes. In some cases it may also be the result of different factors interacting. So, for example, it could be the result of hormonal changes made worse by lack of support, a 'difficult' baby, feeling that you have lost your independence, or motherhood not living up to your expectations. Postnatal depression which emerges a year after the birth is unlikely to be caused by hormonal changes but that doesn't make it any the less real.

The symptoms will also vary a lot from one woman to the next and just because you don't experience the more severe symptoms listed on page 136 it doesn't mean your feelings of depression are any less real or that you shouldn't be 'bothering' your doctor. One of the big hurdles for doctors, midwives and health visitors is to get women to accept that postnatal depression is not something to be ashamed of and kept hidden. You may feel you're being labelled if you accept the diagnosis, but in reality all you are doing is accepting the fact that going through the most incredible physical process imaginable – having a baby – has had an impact on you. And it's very common to feel this way: studies suggest that more than one in ten mothers (and possibly as many as one in five) suffer some form of postnatal depression.

Your health visitor may ask you to complete a questionnaire (called the Edinburgh Postnatal Depression Scale) around the time of your postnatal check. The questionnaire asks you about your feelings over the past week. It's very important to answer the questions honestly: don't try to put on a brave face when help is being offered.

Getting help

The most important thing about postnatal depression is that someone recognizes the symptoms – this person may not be you – and that you accept help from someone who is qualified to counsel or treat you and from all the people around you who want to offer support, friendship and a listening ear. Without help you could struggle for years, not enjoying your baby or your life and missing out. Some women never realize they have postnatal depression until one day – years later – they wake up and feel better. There's no need for it to be like that, although there's no denying it takes courage to admit you need help, particularly if you are a strong person who 'copes' well, if this baby was long-awaited or if everyone around you seems to be managing.

If you think you may be suffering from postnatal depression and you don't feel able to speak to your GP or health visitor about it, then you can get anonymous help from the Association for Postnatal Illness,* a network of volunteers who have suffered and recovered from postnatal depression.

Treatments

- counselling (talking and listening)
- antidepressants
- progesterone injections
- oestrogen patches

Many women with postnatal depression recover within a few months and most are better within twelve to eighteen months, but some suffer for years if they don't get help. Recovery is usually gradual but one day you'll realize it's over and you can move on.

Remember that postnatal depression doesn't necessarily occur in the first few months: some women find it comes later on and sometimes coincides with giving up breastfeeding. Others find the reverse (see story below).

> Ruth developed postnatal depression when her son William was eight weeks old: *'I was in total despair. I felt I couldn't cope and I just sat and cried all the time. I was near to tears in the most ordinary situations and my husband just didn't know what to do with me. We thought it was part of having a child really and I just put up with it until William was about twenty weeks old and I stopped breastfeeding. Things improved then, I presume because the hormones balanced out.'* But the depression returned after Ruth's second child, Emily, was born: *'This time I did the Edinburgh questionnaire and after she'd marked my sheet the health visitor was round and it all came out. My GP prescribed antidepressants which I've been on now for three and a half months. It took nearly three weeks for them to work and at first I felt very detached from everything. One day I watched William pour toys all over the lounge floor and it didn't bother me. That was lovely! That's worn off a bit and I'm more able to think ahead now.*
>
> *'I'm hoping to start reducing the dose in a couple of weeks and then I'll stop altogether and see how things are. My GP thinks the depression was triggered by a hormone imbalance and that things should have settled down by the time Emily is six months old. It'll be interesting to see what happens. I wonder whether it will make a big difference because I'm not sure what effect they're having. My husband said the other day I was much more like my old self and I wasn't at all like myself when I was depressed. It's easy to*

What about my hormones?

assume that's down to the tablets but hopefully my hormones are settling as well.'

Caroline recalls how she realized she had postnatal depression when her daughter Lucy was about three months old: *'My husband Phil was away a lot, and by that time all your help's disappeared. Phil's mum was meant to be coming up but she couldn't and I said, "Don't worry, I can get by." But Lucy wasn't sleeping and she was feeding all the time, and then one night I rang Phil at one o'clock in the morning and just cried and cried. When I spoke to him again later I cried again and he said, "You know what's wrong, don't you?" I went and talked to the GP who was brilliant – gave me a cuddle – but the support I got was useless. The health visitor who came round just wanted me to fill in a form and kept avoiding the issue by talking about Lucy when I wanted to talk about me. It was hopeless. I was crying all the time and at night the loneliness was unbearable: I just kept thinking, "I'm the only person up. Everyone else is asleep." I got through it because I met up with a woman who'd been to my parentcraft classes and she was feeling the same. We just used to talk to each other and it really helps to know you're not the only one. I have to say it took me completely by surprise. When the teacher talked about it at antenatal classes I just thought, "Yes, well, that won't happen to me, this is a very wanted baby," and I threw all the leaflets she gave us away. If I'd met someone who'd had postnatal depression and was prepared to talk about it I might have been more realistic. Women should be more open about it.'*

'Everything seemed like a mountain to climb. I lost all interest in the baby and looking after him became a great chore.'

'It was like a great black cloud over me from the day he was born. I remember looking into the cot and thinking, "So that's it, is it?" It wasn't until I had my second child that I realized what people meant about it being so exciting. It's funny because I'm the last person you'd think would get depressed — it just isn't in my character at all.'

Checklist: symptoms of postnatal depression

Are you suffering from . . .?

- loss of appetite or overeating
- strong feelings of inadequacy, guilt, worthlessness and self-loathing
- feeling sad all the time and crying easily
- lacking energy and enthusiasm; feeling exhausted
- insomnia
- being unable to concentrate – as though you are in a fog
- anxiety, irritability, tension, agitation and panic attacks
- unexpected rage or anger
- feeling neutral or negative towards the baby
- fearing you will harm the baby
- being over-anxious about the baby – showing extreme fear or anxiety
- fussing over the baby without eye contact or love
- hiding feelings because of shame at being depressed
- avoiding seeing people
- non-stop physical problems such as aches and pains

What about my hormones?

Depression self-help

- Don't bottle up your feelings: talk to someone regularly about the way you feel.
- Make time for yourself without the baby each day.
- Eat well: if you don't feel like preparing meals, eat fruit, raw vegetables and cheese.
- Get as much help with housework as possible.
- Keep a diary of your feelings.
- Exercise – swimming and yoga are particularly relaxing.
- Use aromatherapy oils (see page 141).

Q&A

Do I need antidepressants?
A study published in 1997 showed that counselling is as effective as antidepressants for women with postnatal depression, so in one sense, the choice is yours. In practice you may not be offered counselling – because it isn't available or because it might cost more than antidepressants. But lots of women are reluctant to take antidepressants, and with heavyweight research supporting counselling, you're well within your rights to press your GP to find some for you.

I often feel miserable and that I can't cope, but I don't think I've got postnatal depression – what can I do?
Tell your GP, health visitor, antenatal teacher or someone else you trust who will be able to get you some help if you need it.

Not only is it hard to admit you're depressed but many of us simply can't see the signs in ourselves. We're also very good at covering up and putting on a brave face. In one study of women with postnatal depression, only one in three believed they had the condition, although nine out of ten recognized there was something wrong. Eight out of ten hadn't reported their symptoms to a health professional. It doesn't make any sense to go on feeling miserable or desperate. Tell someone today.

Do hormone treatments for PND really work?
The jury is still out on this one. Many doctors aren't convinced there's a hormonal basis to postnatal depression and so far the research has been conflicting. However, a fairly recent study found that women suffering from severe postnatal depression did get better after using oestrogen patches, including some women who hadn't got better using antidepressants.

I feel as though I haven't recovered emotionally from the birth – I keep going over and over in my mind what happened. Will this get better in time?
It may do, but it may not. Having a baby is a major physical and emotional experience. It's hardly surprising if some women are left feeling shocked by what has happened – particularly if they were unprepared, uncertain about what was happening or deeply disappointed by their experience. Sometimes this shock may lead to depression. For example, women having emergency Caesarean sections are more than six times as likely to suffer from postnatal depression as women giving birth vaginally. It's also thought that a few women may suffer a form of 'post traumatic stress disorder' (PTSD) after giving birth. The symptoms of PTSD are flashbacks, nightmares, panic attacks, difficulty sleeping and depression.

What about my hormones?

Even if you don't feel this bad, it often helps if you have the chance to talk to someone about what happened to you when your baby was born, particularly if that person is able to explain some of the events. This can still be helpful even if it takes place months after the birth. You could ask your health visitor or GP to get you an appointment with the consultant in charge of your care at the hospital, or you could arrange to see your community midwife. If you went to antenatal classes then the group leader may be able to help.

Since having my baby I've suffered from really bad PMS – is there a connection?
There could be because your hormones have basically had a shake-up. Some research has suggested that women recovering from postnatal depression suffer relapses in the form of premenstrual syndrome (PMS), even if they never had PMS before (see page 143).

My menstrual cycle has changed since I had my baby – when will it get back to normal?
It's quite common to find that the pattern of your periods changes after you have a baby. They may be more or less regular and more or less heavy. In time they may get back to their previous pattern but many women find the new pattern is the one that lasts.

I stopped breastfeeding two months ago and I still haven't had a period. Is that normal?
It partly depends how long ago your baby was born and how much you were breastfeeding. Women who don't breastfeed fully usually have their first period two or four months after the

baby is born. If your baby is now more than four or five months old, however, and you haven't breastfed at all for two months, it is probably worth seeing your GP. The hormone problems which cause absence of periods (amenorrhoea) are usually easy to correct.

Prozac

One of the newer drugs used to treat postnatal depression is fluoxetine – more commonly known as Prozac. This is a non-addictive drug but it does have some unpleasant side-effects in some women, including nausea, vomiting, diarrhoea and weight loss as well as nervousness and anxiety. Small amounts of Prozac do pass into breastmilk and some doctors suggest you should stop breastfeeding if you want to take it, although it isn't thought to harm the baby. Prozac needs two weeks to take effect.

Many other antidepressants are also used for postnatal depression: if your doctor prescribes one, make sure you get an information sheet with the tablets explaining how long they will take to work and the possible side-effects, including any possible problems with breastfeeding.

Puerperal psychosis

This is a very rare but very serious mental illness which involves hallucinations, delusions, bizarre behaviour and other dramatic personality changes. It usually comes in the first few weeks

What about my hormones?

after childbirth and should be unmistakable. A woman with puerperal psychosis needs to be treated in hospital immediately.

Placenta power

Some people suggest that eating the placenta can ward off or even treat postnatal depression because it contains a wide variety of vitamins and minerals.

> Mary was aware she had an increased risk of having postnatal depression because she had suffered depression in the past, so she decided to save her placenta: 'I remembered reading an article about it and it was quite easy to do as I had a home birth. It was put in a casserole dish and my Mum cut it up and put it in the freezer. She said it was a bit like cutting liver but there was no smell. I didn't need it for the first five weeks but then I started to get depressed and so I started eating inch-square pieces cut up, fried in olive oil and added to my main meal. It lasted about two or three months. It was quite tough, I suppose, and I used to be quite squeamish, but after giving birth you're not so funny about things! It just seemed the sensible thing to do. Has it worked? Well, I've avoided anti depressants so far and the last month without it has been okay.'

Aromatherapy

There are several aromatherapy oils which may help to lift your mood, calm you down and help you sleep. You could put a few drops of the following in the bath, in a burner or on a handkerchief to sniff.

- clary sage: uplifting, relaxing, sedative
- geranium: antidepressant
- lavender: calming, sedative
- marjoram: calming, sedative
- ylang ylang: antidepressant, relaxing

Some aromatherapists suggest you should change the oils you are using after a couple of weeks because you get used to them. So you could try clary sage and geranium followed by ylang ylang and marjoram, or you could try shifting the balance of the mixture to create a slightly different smell. The same oils can be used in massage, but make sure you dilute the oil properly in a carrier oil: some undiluted essential oils can damage your skin. If you are pregnant, breastfeeding, suffer from epilepsy or are taking any prescribed medication, always consult a registered aromatherapist* before choosing your oils.

> Ann used aromatherapy to help counter her depression when she had to return to work just four months after her son was born: 'It was just too soon for me and I couldn't face going back. I didn't have severe depression,' she explains, 'but I got very upset if I tried to talk about it and I was really miserable, weepy and tired. I just couldn't be bothered with anything. My GP recommended I try aromatherapy but I didn't know which oils to use. Fortunately a friend of my mother is an aromatherapist and she recommended I use clary sage and geranium oil. I used to put drops in the bath and burn them in a burner at the same time. That's more or less all I did and after a couple of weeks I felt much better. I still use them now when I feel low.'

What about my hormones?

PMS self-help

Whether it is caused by a hormone imbalance or not, PMS can be a nightmare for you and your family. The symptoms of PMS include fatigue, headache, backache, irritability, mood swings, weight gain, skin eruptions, food cravings, feelings of bloatedness and sore breasts – usually in the ten days or so before a period. Some women have found the following helpful:

- exercise
- evening primrose oil capsules (not to be used with antidepressants)
- eating bread or crackers as snacks (rather than sweets) to satisfy carbohydrate cravings
- aromatherapy – using oils in the bath, in burners or for massage (see above)
- keeping a diary of symptoms – if you can work out when you are likely to be moody or tired you may be able to plan your life around it

Going on the Pill or having specific hormone treatment may also help, but the hormone activity in PMS is very complicated and it could take time to get the right medication. Contact the National Association for Premenstrual Syndrome* for further information.

> Susie didn't suffer from PMS until she stopped breastfeeding her second daughter, Lily: *'I suddenly found I was getting into real rages with the girls – shouting and screaming at them and then collapsing into tears. And there were some days when I was completely exhausted. It took me a long time to realize what was going on: I thought I was a terrible mother and that I just couldn't cope with two children. I can't*

remember why I suddenly thought it could be PMS – perhaps I read something or heard someone mention it on the radio. But after that I started to keep a note of when it happened and there definitely was a pattern. I mentioned it casually in the park one day and both the women I was with said exactly the same thing had happened to them after their second babies were born. Then when I mentioned it to another friend she said she'd been to the doctor's the previous week and been advised to try evening primrose oil. Eventually it seemed that virtually every woman I knew was suffering – and no one had said anything! I tried the evening primrose oil and I think it did work. I stopped after a few months and found things weren't so bad. Now it's limited to about a week in the middle of my cycle and at least I know it's happening, so I try to make sure I have lots of relaxing baths, go to bed early and limit the time I'm on my own with the children.'

Further Information

Helpful organizations

Alexander Technique
See the *Society of Teachers of the Alexander Technique*

Aquaflex (vaginal cones)
Tel: 0800 526177

Aromatherapists
See the *Register of Qualified Aromatherapists* and the *Tisserand Institute of Aromatherapy*

Association for Postnatal Illness (APNI)
25 Jerden Place, Fulham, London SW6 1BE
Tel: 0171 386 0868
10am–5pm, Monday–Friday and 24-hour answerphone
A network of volunteers who have suffered and recovered from postnatal depression themselves and who are willing to support other women.

Birth Crisis Network
Tel: 01865 300266
Help if you need to talk about a difficult birth.

Breastfeeding counsellors
See *Breastfeeding Network*, *La Leche League* and *National Childbirth Trust*

The Breastfeeding Network
PO Box 11126, Paisley PA2 8YB
Breastfeeding counsellors and information.

British Association for Sexual and Marital Therapy
PO Box 13686, London SW20 9ZH
Can provide a list of local therapists.

British Chiropractic Association
29 Whitley Street, Reading RG2 0EG
Tel: 01734 757557

British DSP Support Group
17 Muir Road, Dumpton, Ramsgate, Kent CT11 8AX
Tel: 01843 587356

British Homeopathic Association
27a Devonshire Street, London W1N 1RJ
Tel: 0171 935 2163
Provides a list of medically qualified doctors who are also qualified in homeopathy, as well as pharmacists who stock homeopathic medicines.

Chiropractors
See *British Chiropractic Association*

Further Information

Continence Foundation
307 Hatton Square, 16 Baldwins Gardens, London EC1N 7RJ
Tel: 0171 831 9831
9.30am–5.30pm, Monday–Friday
Information and confidential help.

General Council and Register of Osteopaths
56 London Street, Reading, Berkshire RG1 4SQ
Tel: 01734 576585
Provides a list of registered osteopaths.

Herbalists
See the *National Institute of Medical Herbalists*

Homeopaths
See the *British Homeopathic Association* and the *Society of Homeopaths*

La Leche League
BM 3424, London WC1N 3XX
Tel: 0171 242 1278
Support for breastfeeding mothers.

Meet-A-Mum Association (MAMA)
26 Avenue Road, London SE25 4DX
Tel: 0181 771 5595
Puts you in touch with other mums in your area.

National Association for Premenstrual Syndrome (NAPS)
PO Box 72, Sevenoaks, Kent TN13 1XQ
Tel: 01732 459378
For sufferers of PMS and postnatal depression.

National Back Pain Association
16 Elmtree Road, Teddington TW11 8ST
Tel: 0181 977 5474

National Childbirth Trust (NCT)
Alexandra House, Oldham Terrace, Acton, London W3 6NH
Tel: 0181 992 8637
9.30am–4.30pm, Monday–Friday
Antenatal classes, breastfeeding counsellors, postnatal discussion groups, national experience register, friendship with other parents and local support groups including support after a Caesarean.

NCT Maternity Sales
239 Shawbridge Street, Glasgow G43 1QN
Tel: 0141 636 0600
Feeding bras, stretch briefs and other items for sale. Your local branch of the NCT (see above) may have a local MAVA bra agent who can measure you for a feeding bra.

The National Institute of Medical Herbalists
56 Longbrook Street, Exeter EX4 6AH
Tel: 01392 426022.
Provides a list of qualified practitioners.

National Osteoporosis Society
PO Box 10, Radstock, Bath BA3 3YB
Tel: 01761 471771. Helpline: 01761 472721
Produces a booklet on osteoporosis in pregnancy.

Osteopathic Information Service
4 Harcourt House, 19a Cavendish Square, London W1M 9AD

Further Information

List of registered practitioners.
(See also *General Council and Register of Osteopaths*)

Register of Qualified Aromatherapists
Tel: 01245 227957
Will send a list of aromatherapists in your area who have been trained to an approved standard (usually one or two years of training).

Relate
(Look in the phone book for details of your local branch.)
Sexual and relationship counselling.

Society of Homeopaths
2 Artizan Road, Northampton NN1 4HU.
Tel: 01604 21400

Society of Teachers of the Alexander Technique
20 London House, 266 Fulham Road, London SW10 9EL
Tel: 0171 351 0828

Tisserand Institute of Aromatherapy
Tel: 01273 206640
Names and telephone numbers for aromatherapists in your area who have done the Tisserand Diploma in Aromatherapy.

Vaginal cones
See *Aquaflex*

Weight Watchers
Tel: 01628 777077
All enquiries about local classes.

Useful books and videos

Aromatherapy Massage Book by Clare Maxwell-Hudson (Dorling Kindersley, £9.99)

Caesarean Birth – Your Questions Answered by Debbie Chippington Derrick, Gina Lowden and Fiona Barlow (NCT Maternity Sales, £3.50)

Get into Shape after Childbirth by Gillian Fletcher (Ebury Press, £9.99)

Is There Sex after Childbirth? by Juliet Rix (Thorsons, £7.99).

The BBC Pregnancy and Postnatal Exercise Video with Rosemary Conley and Jane Ashton (BBC, £10.99)

The Caesarean Experience by Dr Sarah Clement (Pandora, £7.99)

The Postnatal Exercise Book by M. Polden and B. Whitford (Frances Lincoln, £7.99)

Women's Waterworks – Curing Incontinence by Pauline E. Chiarelli (NCT Maternity Sales, £4.95)